Nature's Sports Pharmacy

A NATURAL APPROACH TO PEAK ATHLETIC PERFORMANCE

Frederick C. Hatfield, Ph.D.,
and Frederick C. Hatfield II, M.S.

CB

CONTEMPORARY BOOKS

Library of Congress Cataloging-in-Publication Data

Hatfield, Frederick C.
    Nature's sports pharmacy : a natural approach to peak athletic performance /
Frederick C. Hatfield and Frederick C. Hatfield II.
      p.   cm.
    Includes bibliographical references and index.
    ISBN 0-8092-3221-9
    1. Sports medicine.   2. Herbs—Therapeutic use.   I. Hatfield, Frederick C., II.
II. Title.
RC1210.H32   1999
613.7′11—dc20   96-1350
                                                              CIP

Also by Frederick C. Hatfield, Ph.D.

Bodybuilding: A Scientific Approach

Hardcore Bodybuilding: A Scientific Approach

Power: A Scientific Approach

Ultimate Sports Nutrition:
A Scientific Approach to Peak Athletic Performance

Illustrations on pp. 60 and 90 courtesy of Odyssey International
and Lifetech Resources, LLC
Cover design by Todd Petersen
Cover photograph copyright © 1998 Kurt Gerber
Cover photograph model: Martin Berke
Interior design by Jeanette Wojtyla

Published by Contemporary Books
A division of NTC/Contemporary Publishing Group, Inc.
4255 West Touhy Avenue, Lincolnwood (Chicago), Illinois 60646-1975 U.S.A.
Copyright © 1999 by Fred Hatfield
Printed in the United States of America
International Standard Book Number: 0-8092-3221-9

99 00 01 02 03 04 QV 20 19 18 17 16 15 14 13 12 11 10 9 8 7 6 5 4 3 2 1

Kristen, my lovely teenager-to-be little big girl, shows signs of athletic greatness. She made the All-Stars four years running in softball. Beau, my youngest son, is known by all for his strong yet tender spirit. It is because of this admirable quality that he too shall become great. It is to them that I dedicate this work. If ever there were two youngsters deserving of a father's love and praise, she's that little girl and he's that little boy. All that I do I do for them.

Frederick C. Hatfield

I would like to thank my family for all the love and support they have given me over the years. Special thanks goes to E. J. "Doc" Kreis of the University of Colorado, Matt Riley of Middle Tennessee State University, Greg Werner of James Madison University, Bob Otrando of the University of Massachusetts, and the great staff at the International Sports Sciences Association. These people are my mentors and provided expert guidance to me through the difficult years while I was developing my philosophy of sports conditioning. I would especially like to extend my appreciation to the many athletes whom I have trained over the years, each as much a teacher to me as I was to them.

Frederick C. Hatfield II

Contents

Introduction

Over the many years that we have been associated with the sports nutrition industry, we have seen various substances purported to provide near magical increases in muscle development, strength, fat loss, and health. They've all come and gone. None has held a candle to the awesome power of herbs or extracted herb-based phytochemicals. Indeed, there is a powerful trend growing stronger each day in the sports nutrition industry toward the use of herbs.

Not too long ago there was no such thing as "drugs." Throughout the history of mankind well into the twentieth century, medical practitioners relied on the bounties Mother Nature provided for their curative potions. Every species of flowers, roots, fruits, leaves, bark—even microscopic algae—had long since been exploited by the ancients for their medicinal properties.

But the exploitation of Earth's botanical bounty was not limited to medicine. No indeed! Humans, you see, have always been ascendant in their thinking. They want *more* than they are born with. They want greater powers of concentration, stronger muscles, heightened awareness, and keener survival skills of various sorts. And they want to have fun—to play and to make sport.

The wherewithal both to improve themselves and their lot in life and to engage in sporting endeavors has, since time immemorial, been amplified and supported by powerful substances contained in the plant life of this world. Botanicals—"herbal medicines"—are our gift from the Creator. That they are effective is self-evident. Millennia of use and thousands upon thousands of research projects give testament to this fact. The vast majority of today's powerful drugs are directly botanical in origin.

No one in history has ever pulled the best herbal substances together into a coherent, integrated system for use in sports. No one, that is, until now. The future of sports nutrition may well be grounded in the wisdom of the past. Powerful and effective herbs have always been here, and they are here to stay so long as people aspire to excel.

Disclaimer

This book is intended for informational use only. The information contained here is based on various published and unpublished sources. It represents training, fitness, health, nutrition, and herbal literature and practice as summarized by the authors. The publisher of this book makes no warranties, expressed or implied, regarding the currency, completeness, or scientific accuracy of this information, nor does it endorse the information for any particular purpose. The information is not intended for use in connection with the sale of any product. Any claims or presentations regarding any specific products or brand names are strictly the responsibility of the product owners or manufacturers. This summary of information from unpublished sources, books, research journals, and articles is not intended to replace the advice or attention of health-care professionals. It is not intended to direct their behavior or replace their independent professional judgment. If you have a problem with your health, or before you embark on any health, fitness, or sports-training program, seek clearance from a qualified health-care professional.

Some herbs can trigger allergic reactions in sensitive people or produce discomfort or illness if taken in excess. Also, many herbs have secondary actions which may be medically contraindicated or in some way counterproductive to your training objectives. Potential side effects of some herbs include diarrhea, cramping, blurred vision, dilated pupils, dry mouth, disorientation, liver toxicity, high blood pressure, tremor, and irritability. Allergic reactions have also been reported. Some of these allergic reactions may not develop immediately but occur after prolonged use of a certain substance.

Amendments to the 1938 Federal Food, Drug, and Cosmetic Act require that all drugs marketed in the United States after 1962 be proven both safe and effective. However, most herbal products are not classified as drugs. They are sold and distributed in retail stores under the categories of herbs, teas, health foods, food supplements, and nutritional and natural products. Therefore, they are considered food products and are not subject to scrutiny at this time.

Many herbal preparations contain substances which are banned from use in sport. One example is ma huang, or Chinese ephedra, the naturally occurring plant containing the banned stimulant substance ephedrine. Some examples of products that have been known to contain ma huang, or ephedra, are Bishop's Tea, Brigham Tea, Chi Powder, Energy Rise, Ephedra Excel, Joint Fir, Mexican Tea, Popotillo, Squaw Tea, Super Charge, and Teamster's Tea.

Many herbal products also have diuretic actions. Diuretics are a class of drugs banned by the U.S. Olympic Committee (USOC) and the International Olympic Committee (IOC). Common examples of herbs with diuretic actions include lily of the valley, sarsaparilla, uva ursi, and horsetail. Use of such herbs with diuretic properties can dilute the urine and result in mandatory detention for athletes during drug testing.

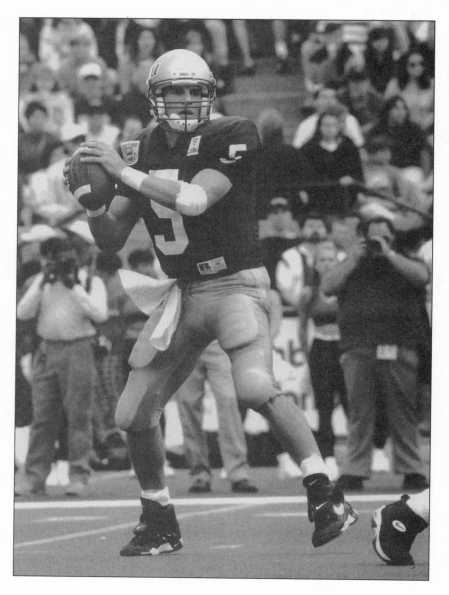

People have always wanted more than they were born with. They want greater powers of concentration, stronger muscles, heightened awareness, and keener survival skills. And they want to have fun—to play and make sport.

I

A Brief Overview of Herbalism

*"Herbalism is an ancient and venerable art that has thrived in
all cultures of the world and in all historical periods, until the
very recent past in the industrialized West. As a constant and
vital thread in human life, it is alive and well and even in the
western world there is a rediscovery of the value of herbal
medicine. The rich and colorful history of herbalism is the
history of humanity itself. As a branch of medicine it has
occasionally found itself on the wrong side of the establishment,
but this ebb & flow of acceptance is just an artifact of the
changing fashions and opinions of medical and legal elites."*
—*David Hoffman,* **The Herbalist**

People have used herbs for more than sixty thousand years. Yet in
the past hundred years, since the advent of the drug age, herbs have
been all but abandoned as viable medications by medical practitioners, especially in the United States. This does not mean that
herbs are of no use to you as an athlete. On the contrary, there
appears to be a newfound interest in the healing power of herbs just
beginning in the United States, although it's not the medical practitioners who are showing interest. Instead, it's laypeople: athletes,
fitness buffs, health freaks. You and me. Self-taught herbalists are
growing in number, much to the dismay of those formally schooled
in herbalism. We believe this interest will continue to grow particularly among athletes who have always sought an edge for improved
performance ability. That's why we—self-taught "performance
herbalists"—are writing this book.

1

The earliest record of medicinal exploitation of herbs goes back sixty thousand years to a grave discovered by archeologists in northern Iraq. They found what appeared to be a Neanderthal medicine man surrounded by the remains of eight species of flowers, most of which are used to this day by the inhabitants of the region.

Ayurveda, sometimes referred to as the world's oldest health-care system, originated in India more than five thousand years ago. While much of this knowledge is believed to have been lost over the centuries, a vast record of precise and sophisticated applications for thousands of herbs has been recorded, largely through the efforts of the Maharishi Mahesh Yoga, a famous modern-day seer.

An Egyptian papyrus document written more than thirty-five hundred years ago lists nearly seven hundred herbal remedies, many of which are still used today. And, somewhat later than Ayurveda, written records that document the practice of Sumerian and Chinese herbalism have been dated to sometime between the year 2000 B.C. and 2700 B.C. The Sumerian record was thought to be written by an herbalist named Enlil-bani. Noted herbs in this book include laurels, still used today for digestive disorders as well as colds and flu; caraway, used to help menstruation and cramps; and thyme, used to soothe coughs, sore throats, swelling, and bruises. All are still recommended by herbalists today.

Shen-Nung, a Chinese emperor, is believed to be the first herbalist to record herbs used for medical purposes in a document known as *Pen Tsao*, which was written around 2700 B.C. Huang-Ti, another emperor, wrote *Nei Ching Su Wen* sometime around 2600 B.C. Among the herbs discussed was ma huang, still used today to produce ephedrine and widely used by athletes despite being on the IOC's list of banned ergogens (substances with known performance-enhancing properties).

The American Indians, Mayans, Aztecs, and Incas also had a sophisticated herb-based healing system. In fact, most cultures throughout history are known to have used indigenous plants as medicine. The ancients regarded herbs as being so powerful that they often worshipped them as gods.

The Chinese philosophy of treating illness, along with that of Eastern Indians, Tibetans, and American Indians, greatly differs from how we treat illness in the United States today. While we try to isolate the disease or symptoms from the person and then treat the disease by relieving symptoms, the philosophy of these ancient cultures is to treat the underlying cause of the disease. While we tend to take aspirin for a headache, the philosophy of these ancient cultures is to try to cure what caused the headache in the first place.

The current drug-based—or allopathic—medical philosophy and use of chemical drugs came about for several reasons. A paradigm shift of major proportions taking place at the beginning of the industrial revolution spawned a reductionist point of view among many industries, including medicine. Scientists were, for the first time ever, able to isolate specific elements and break complex chemical compounds down into their component parts.

But let's get real for a moment. Because of these major advancements in both science and technology, *money* became the major force in shaping current allopathic medical philosophy. As chemical medicines became more popular—and profitable for pharmaceutical companies—herbal medicines declined to the point of being known as "old wives' tales" or "folk medicine." The first big blow to herbalism and naturopathy (which combines the use of herbs with healthy living practices) came in 1910 with the publication of the *Flexnor Report*, which was a survey distributed to medical schools to find those willing to develop and research chemical drugs in exchange for financial aid. Since these subjects were not of high interest to naturopaths or herbalists, they did not participate, they lost financial backing, and the vast majority of their schools were closed.

Herbs and Peak Athletic Performance

It is not our intent to talk about the use of herbs for curing or preventing disease; to do so would be a foolish replication of the work hundreds of brilliant herbalists have done so very well already. What we want to talk about is sports. But consider that the need to perform optimally while maintaining good health was a critical element of our ancient forebears. And in fact, hardworking humans bent on surviving were conditioned much in the same way that today's athletes are. They ran, they jumped, they fought, and they pulled and pushed against rocks, brush, and game for food, clothes, and shelter.

Only recently have humans had little use for physical prowess as a survival skill. In other words, an important difference between our ancient ancestors and athletes of today is that the old-timers were conditioned by their survivalist lifestyles. Today's athletes must actually make a point of getting into shape because their lifestyles are utterly sedentary by comparison!

If you agree with this way of thinking, you will realize that many of the herbs used for centuries by our predecessors went far beyond providing health and preventing disease. In earlier times, if you got sick, you would either die or get better fast. Your life depended on being in optimal health. Healing or recovering quickly was far more critical for survival then than now. So was endurance. So was strength. And so was speed. Indeed, many of the organized sports practiced today mimic the physical skills needed for survival by our forebears. Running, jumping, shooting, fighting, riding. The list goes on. These are the same physical attributes sedentary folks of today have chosen to eschew and ascribe instead to our athletes.

So, throughout this book, we will discuss many herbs and combinations of herbs in light of their potential use by athletes. You may wonder whether an athlete who doesn't use performance-enhancing drugs and only uses herbs would ever be able to run with the "big dogs." We think so. In fact, the minor thrust of this book is to inform you of alternatives to dangerous drugs.

Whether you know it or not, and whether the drug companies like to admit it, herbs have always been—and still are—a vital part of your health and nutrition. More to the point, they are also quite relevant to the needs of athletes seeking peak performance capabilities.

It's clear that herbs just need to be rediscovered for their ergogenic properties as they are beginning to be for their medicinal ones. While there is much solid scientific evidence documenting the use of herbs for good health and longevity, not a lot has been written about the use of herbs specifically for the purpose of improving or maximizing athletic performance, which is rather strange considering that almost all ancient societies had athletes and athletic competitions. Ancient athletes were revered then as they are today—remember, the Greeks gave much social status to their Olympians. However, these societies didn't document their training methods to any significant degree. From what we do know, sporting competition was a reflection of their society; skills in sport were similar to those used in battle and hunting. It is easy to see how wrestling, running, archery, the biathlon, the javelin, and the martial arts all became competitive sports in ancient society. These sports contained the very skills of survival that the athletes used in their daily lives! But in modern times, we have separated athletic performance from survival.

To see how athletes in history have used nature's sports pharmacy to enhance their athletic performance, whether to improve overall health or to win the olive wreath, we should look at the herbs they used to develop such skills. Which herbs made them run faster? Which herbs improved endurance? How did they increase strength through herbs? What made them tough enough to face a raging bull in an enclosed arena? Whatever it was, *citius, altius, fortius* (faster, higher, stronger) was as much a slogan then as now among sportsmen.

Used by Ancient Athletes

The ancient Sumerians wrote about a mixture of laurels, thyme, and caraway. These herbs, while enhancing digestive properties and appetite, can also help reduce swelling and sprains. Throughout the centuries, and even today, these herbs have been used for the same purpose, especially among athletes. Ancient Chinese herbalists documented more than 300 herbs that could have been used for vitality. Ma huang, which even today is popular (though banned) as a peak performance aid, was used to treat headaches, colds, and fevers. The alkaloid found in ma huang, or ephedra, raises your heart rate, which gives the illusion of increased energy. Other herbs used for increased energy included astragalus, codonopsis, dioscorea, ginseng, schizandra, and zizyphus (all of which are commonly available today).

Other herbs were used to strengthen many other functions related to athletic performance in ancient China, including aconite for pain relief, low metabolism, and nervousness; dong quai for blurred vision and injuries; fu ling for anxiety; honeysuckle for inflammation and swelling; pueraria for muscle pain and tightness; reishi for fatigue, stress, and weakness (today it's sometimes used to treat cancer and AIDS); and tien qi or tienchi for injury and wounds.

Performance-Enhancement Herbs Used by Modern Athletes

Despite the dearth of hard evidence, it is not unreasonable to speculate that athletes in ancient cultures used herbs, even while they were otherwise healthy. More recently, athletes from the former Soviet Union used herbs extensively in their training and contest preparation. Dr. Ben Tabachnik, former head of the Scientific Research Group for the Soviet National Track and Field Team, described the use of herbs, especially adaptogens, by athletes in the former Soviet Union:

> The use of plant- and animal-based adaptogens by Soviet athletes is a common practice. Western athletes on the other hand approach herbal preparations with much skepticism. They have been led to believe natural medicines are not as effective as synthetic drugs. This is a great error, and western athletes have missed out on a classification of sport pharmacology that is safe and effective.
>
> Adaptogens are prescribed by Soviet sports physicians to athletes in order to prepare them for an enormous amount of work during high-load training cycles. Soviet coaches recognize that the more an athlete trains, the more he or she has a chance of winning high level competitions, so they train them very hard. From one training session to the next the athlete must replenish depleted structural and psychological reserves.

The Soviets had found that adaptogens like Siberian ginseng and schizandra (berries from a type of magnolia plant) were useful for athletes to adapt to the stress caused by long trips involving jet lag as well as to training and competition stresses.

Of course, an athlete's lifestyle doesn't help matters. Athletes have succumbed to a world of quick fixes resulting from a do-or-die mentality. How often is it heard on the sidelines, "Hey, Doc, I pulled my hamstring. Gimme a shot or something! I gotta finish the game!"

How many athletes routinely go underground to find a black-market source for uppers, anabolic steroids, or painkillers? Sadly, the answer is most of them.

Using drugs in this manner is only a short-term solution to your athletic problems. Herbs, on the other hand, can gently coax your body to adapt to the stresses of training, and give you greater energy, mental focus, and healing powers. Drugs often create side effects or health problems while trying to ameliorate symptoms, whereas the only side effects you're likely to experience with herbs will be improved systemic functioning. However, you should be aware that, just as performance-enhancing drugs are banned by all the sport governing bodies and by federal law, some herbs are so powerful they've been banned as well!

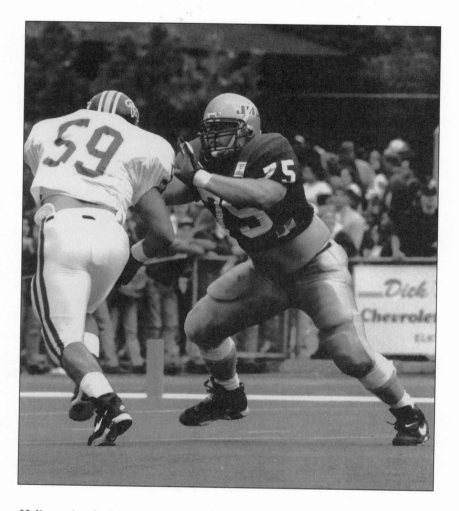

Holism, simply defined, means taking all things into consideration in order to solve a puzzle. Herbalists speak of holism as though they invented the concept. Athletes have been practicing holistic training since time began.

2

Herbal Theory

"Their fruit will be for food, and their leaves for healing."
—*Ezekiel 47:12*

Exactly what is herbalism? A layperson might naively reply, "The study of herbs." This definition is far too vague to really explain the term. Herbalism has been around for more than sixty thousand years, so there has to be more to it than such a short description! For centuries, various permutations of naturopathy, of which herbalism forms an integral part, were the only viable health-care systems. Herbalism has been pushed to the back of the medical texts as a curious and unscientific form of quackery politely referred to as "folk medicine." Forgotten is the foundation herbalism provided for the very basis of modern medicine: botany, pharmacology, and chemistry. Also forgotten by many is the fact that an estimated 75 percent of the drugs used today have botanical origins.

Those with a holistic view of herbalism describe it as our relation to the plant kingdom. Using this definition, we can more clearly visualize how herbs impact our lives. If you stop and think, everything from the wood we use to build our houses and furniture, the threads which make our clothes, the dyes we use for our hair and clothes, the medicine we use, the air we breathe, and the food we eat are donated by ever-generous, patient, uncomplaining plants!

Slowly but steadily, drug-based medical practitioners are realizing that the entire person must be tended to, not just the ailing body part. The old YMCA triangle logo depicting humans as being comprised of a body, a mind, and a spirit was borrowed from the aboriginals of North America. There is no telling how many eons ago this utterly modern concept came to them. One thing is clear— herbal theory embraces this universal understanding of humanity.

Let's focus on the amazing complexity of just one point of the human triangle. Your body. It has been said that no man is an island. Likewise no organ of the body acts independently of the others. For example, just like all the tissues of your body, the brain is dependent on the circulatory system to bring it nutrients and dispose of waste. Without the kidneys and accompanying organs of the urinary system, those wastes would not be removed, and neither your circulatory system nor urinary system could operate without neural impulses initiated by your brain.

It's an utterly complex, integrated circle! All systems are inextricably interrelated. A problem in one organ left untended inevitably comes to bear on the efficient functioning of all others, including the mind. This reality has prompted the World Health Organization (WHO) to redefine the word *health*: "Health is more than simply the absence of illness. It is the active state of physical, emotional, mental, and social well-being."

This new definition, if you give the WHO a bit of slack for leaving out the "spirit" point of the triangle, constitutes a viable definition of life itself, and is the basis of a holistic approach to more than just herbal medicine. Holistic thought dictates that medical treatment should involve the entire body, never focusing on one aspect of health while compromising another. Perhaps David Hoffman in *The Herbalist* put it best: "When the healing process is separated too far from the humanity of the people involved, there is nothing other than chemistry and surgery. The hearts of doctor and patient must meet as well as their skill and symptoms."

As we've discussed, herbs have laid the foundation for modern medicine, as a great majority of the chemical drugs used today have botanical origin. But it goes deeper than that. Herbal theory is heavily oriented toward preventing disease. Proper use of herbs will gently coax your body toward optimal health by having an impact on all of the systems of your body. However, when illness does strike, a holistic application of herbal medicine will treat the cause of your illness rather than merely the symptoms—in a sense, removing the thorn instead of just easing the pain.

Modern medicine seems all too geared to treat the symptoms of disease, injury, and health problems. The doctors aren't the only ones involved either. It is a common human tendency to always be in a hurry. For example, you've probably encountered what you believed to be muscle soreness or stiffness from time to time. Once you got rid of the pain, you could train again or "get back in the game." The problem is your muscle got sore or stiff for a reason. It may have been your body's way of saying, "Hey, the muscle is damaged! Don't do anymore until it's healed!" Did you listen? No, you told it to shut up and get back to work by blocking the pain.

This is an approach not even contemplated in holistic herbalism. Instead, you would use nutrients from herbs as well as proper eating patterns and exercise to clear wastes out of the muscle, increase the capacity of your body's normal healing processes, reduce swelling, increase blood flow, and, yes, even relieve pain. You would also aid the entire holistic process by meditation, normalizing your sleep patterns, increasing your body's anabolic (tissue growth) capacity, reducing its catabolic (tissue destruction) responses, and improving digestive and eliminative functions. In short, you get your whole body and being involved in the healing process! Throw in some ice to reduce inflammation and massage therapy to break up scar tissue and adhesions, and your muscle has fully recovered, stronger than it was before the injury.

Is this a more complicated and lengthy solution than simply popping a few pills? It may seem so. But bear in mind that by falsely relieving the pain you didn't really heal the muscle. In fact, you probably made it worse.

Holistic theory is not restricted to herbalism. Whether you realize it or not, you have probably used this approach in preparing for sports competition. For example, in team sports, for the defense to be effective, it must be ready to counter all offensive possibilities. This basic principle is applied universally in politics, war, teaching, or any other situation where more than one outcome is possible. Maximizing the health of all your body's systems, including your mind and spirit, will lead to optimum sports performance capabilities with no negative side effects. You have, in essence, reduced the number of possible outcomes and improved your chances for success in the process.

Covering all your bases in any sports situation is not easy. The approach you take must work for you within the context of the entire team. Likewise, your approach to health must not cause a strategic breakdown by developing weaknesses and harmful side effects. So, before you plan your holistic approach to herbal use, there are questions that need to be answered.

1. *What effects will the herbs have?* How will the herbs affect the physiology of your entire body? For example, if you are tired and sluggish prior to a competition, you wouldn't want to take valerian root since it tends to have a more calming effect rather than a stimulating effect. Obviously, choice of treatment will depend on accurately identifying the problem, which involves:
   - Using some diagnostic procedure to identify what physiological process must be addressed
   - Selecting appropriate actions to achieve immediate relief
   - Selecting relevant herbs based on their range of primary and secondary actions to ensure the long-term results

2. *What is each herb's affinity?* Some herbs work directly on a specific system, organ, or tissue while others help many or all systems of the body. Such is the case with herbal tonics. For example, a combination of hawthorn and motherwort is beneficial to the actions of the heart while ginseng can aid the entire body.

3. *Which herbs will treat specific problems?* While the holistic approach covers overall health, there are times when specific problems must be addressed. There are many herbs which directly treat a specific illness or injury.

4. *What is the herb's pharmacology?* Knowledge of herbal pharmacology has led to the development of many breakthrough drugs. But this approach tends to isolate one specific phytochemical of the herb and disregard the rest. So, while this is not the holistic approach to herbal use, it should nonetheless be considered and used when appropriate.

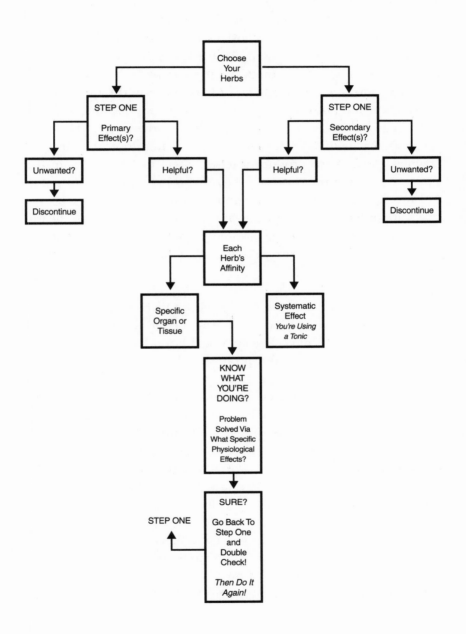

5. *Do you know what you are taking?* Plants have roots, stems, fruit, leaves, and flowers. What's in them, and what part is best? Where is the plant grown? What sort of climate conditions, soil characteristics, and preparation methods are considered optimal or vital? For example, it's the root of the rhubarb plant that's used in herbal preparations; the stem is eaten as food, not used as an herb. All parts of a rhubarb plant contain oxalate crystals as well as anthraquinone glycosides, which reportedly have been the cause of poisoning, but *only* when huge quantities of raw or cooked leaves are ingested. The LD50 (LD50 is the median lethal dose, which is the dose of a drug or chemical *predicted* to produce a lethal effect in 50 percent of the subjects to whom the dose is given) for oxalic acid given to rats is 375 mg/kg. So for a person weighing about 145 pounds (65.7 kg) that's about 25 grams of pure oxalic acid required to cause death. Rhubarb leaves are probably around 0.5% oxalic acid, so that you would need to eat a full 5 kilograms (11 lb.) to get 24 grams of oxalic acid.

6. *Do you know how much to take?* How much of any given herb should you use? Almost all of the herbs cited in this book are readily available in the United States in health food stores (typically in extract or pill form) or from professional herbalists, and they are almost always provided in standardized dosages. All one has to do is follow the directions labeled on the herb container. Since a vast majority of the herbs commonly available in these stores or through herbalists contain no potent or toxic constituents, the issue of safety is practically irrelevant. "Usually, however, dosage is not too critical," says David Hoffman, in *The Herbalist.* "The problem is one of too little being given rather than too much. From my British perspective the doses used in the U.S. are absurdly low . . ."

Still, the danger exists, however small. Guidelines relating to dosage of herbs and proportions in combining herbs are discussed later in this chapter. But the best advice we can give you on the issues of safety, efficacy, and dosages is to check with a qualified herbalist.

Physiological Actions of Herbs

Clearly, modern medicine has made use of the active constituents found in herbs, and scientists continue to study herbs to unlock even more secrets of the actions of various phytochemicals. Cases in point:

- Hypericin, a chemical compound found in St. John's wort, may inhibit some retroviral infections. Its effects are being studied as a possible AIDS medication.
- The National Cancer Institute is researching highly concentrated anticarcinogens found in plants. These designer foods include phytochemicals from certain plants, for example, indoles from cabbage and triterpenoids from licorice.
- In the past 10 years, thousands of studies have been conducted on the anti-aging effects of free-radical scavengers found in vegetables and other plant life. These include proanthocyanidins from the maritime pine tree, catechins found in green tea, and nordihydroguaiaritic acid (NDGA) from chaparral.

Could it be that the plant life on earth has the ability to prevent or cure any ailment? There is no doubt that many of the deepest secrets of Mother Nature have not yet been unlocked. We may indeed find cures for many forms of cancer and for AIDS in plant life. If compounds found in plants are powerful enough to combat deadly diseases, just think what they can do for athletic performance.

Let's back up for a moment and again define just what we mean by the word *herbs.*

An often-used definition of herbs is any part of a plant that can be used as a medical treatment, nutrient, food seasoning, or dye. However, this definition is too shortsighted to be relevant to the needs of otherwise healthy athletes whose major objective is to excel in their respective sports. You can use herbs to enhance your performance in many ways:

- Herbs can add seasoning to bland, low-fat food so commonly eaten by athletes as well as active people interested in maximizing their fitness.
- Herbs can cleanse. Your blood, liver, kidneys, and gastrointestinal tract often need a bit of "housekeeping" in order to improve the functioning of the entire body while under stress or recuperating from stress.
- Many herbs contain powerful antioxidants whose ability to slow the aging process in addition to aiding in recovery has been well documented.
- Herbs can have a normalizing effect, allowing your body to both recuperate from and adapt to the intense stresses of workouts and competition.
- Herbs can have great nutritional value. Many herbs are high in vitamins and minerals which you as an athlete need at higher levels because of your extremely active lifestyle or dietary limitations.
- Herbs can raise your energy levels as well as provide greater endurance.
- Herbs can stimulate your endocrine system, which plays a part in *all* bodily functions, including muscle-tissue repair and growth.

In the past, most herbalists categorized herbs by the actions they have on the body rather than their chemical makeup, although at times they are very similar. This classification system continues to be used by many herbalists.

Action-Based Classes of Herbs

Adaptogens

Adaptogens help the body cope with stress through biochemical support of the adrenal glands. The term *adaptogen* was coined by researchers to describe the action of a substance that helps increase resistance to adverse influences, both physical and environmental—a cure-all. To be a true adaptogen the substance must (1) be safe for daily use, (2) increase the body's resistance to a wide variety of factors, and (3) have a normalizing action in the body. Adaptogens are useful for otherwise healthy individuals to help them adapt to stresses such as an increasing work load, illness, or injury. Adaptogens provide a tonic support to help the body normalize as well as provide primary medical treatment.

Adaptogens work best over time, gently and efficiently coaxing your body into a far more strategic position for maintaining improved growth, recovery, and repair for the months of hard training you are about to enter. The first step is to prepare your body for better use of supplements and dietary intake. This is done using a cleansing formula for your kidneys, liver, colon, and blood. Step two is to improve your body's wound-healing (restorative and recovery) ability. The final step is to maximize your body's adaptive responses to the stresses of training, which involves boosting immune function.

One of the most well known adaptogens is Siberian ginseng. Other herbs such as chaparral, dandelion root, aloe vera, echinacea, yellow dock, and goldenseal also have adaptogenic properties.

Alteratives

Alteratives work by gradually restoring the proper functioning of the body. One main function of alteratives is to neutralize toxins in the blood. Indeed, an alternative name for alteratives is "blood cleansers." But because alteratives also help the kidneys, liver, lungs, skin, and other systems remove toxins with their restorative properties, the term *blood cleanser* is not complete. Some herbs with alterative properties include nettle, cleavers, burdock, dandelion, yellow dock, red clover, chaparral, and Oregon grapes.

Anticatarrhals

Anticatarrhals help your body get rid of excess mucous from the lungs, sinuses, and throat. Athletes engaged in severe aerobic activities or challenged by extreme bouts against the anaerobic threshold (to the point where further movement is impossible without more oxygen being available) are clearly aided by anticatarrhal herbs such as goldenrod, elder tree, and eyebright.

Anti-inflammatories

Anti-inflammatories reduce swelling in various bodily tissues. Most herbs with anti-inflammatory properties contain volatile oils. These herbs can work by relaxing the nervous system and muscle spasms, attacking bacteria, or by increasing blood flow to the affected area. In doing so, the herb may also relieve pain. This is clearly a category of herbs of extreme interest to athletes. Remember, no healing or recovery is possible until you first reduce swelling and inflammation. Some herbs with anti-inflammatory properties include chamomile, lemon balm, peppermint, meadowsweet, willow bark, bog bean, and wild yams.

Antimicrobials and Antibacterials

Micro-organisms and bacteria can disrupt the body's systems and cause illness. By stimulating the body's immune system, or by direct attack, antimicrobials and antibacterials keep these pathogens at bay. Chaparral, echinacea, garlic, and goldenseal are herbs with excellent antimicrobial and antibacterial actions.

Antispasmodics

Antispasmodics relieve muscle cramps by alleviating muscular tension, nervous tension, or psychological tension. This is another class of herbs offering great benefit for athletes. Black haw, grindelia, lobelia, angelica, and peppermint all have antispasmodic properties.

Astringents

Astringents tighten or bond tissues together by binding protein molecules, causing contraction and firming of tissues. This effect is useful for cuts or abrasions, sinusitis, and diarrhea. Herbs with an astringent property include white oak, pipsissewa, horse chestnut, witch hazel, agrimony, and cranesbill.

Bitters

Bitters got their name not by what they do but by how they taste— yet it is the taste that helps the body detoxify itself. The bitter sensation triggers a hormonal response in the digestive system that leads to the production of digestive juices and bile, as well as detoxification of the liver. Athletes having a hard time gaining weight because of poor appetite or poor digestion can benefit greatly from the use of bitters before each of their five to six daily meals. Bitters can also stimulate intestinal healing. Herbs with bitter properties include gentian, citrus peel, angelica, barberry, burdock, dandelion, mugwort, horehound, elecampane, turmeric, and ginseng.

Calmatives and Carminatives

The aromatic volatile oils found in calmatives reduce inflammation in the intestinal walls. By doing this, they promote proper functioning of the digestive system, relieve intestinal pain, and remove gas. Calmatives' effects on the digestive system will promote better nutrients absorption as well as help relieve pre-competition upset stomach. Fennel and rosemary are a couple of herbs that have calmative effects.

Like calmatives, carminatives have a strong effect on the digestive system. They ease gas, indigestion, intestinal cramping, and can also stimulate appetite. Cumin, fennel, ginger, and peppermint are a few carminatives.

Demulcents

When the kidneys and bladder become irritated, proper waste elimination is compromised. The mucous membranes found in the throat and nasal cavity also can become inflamed, dry, and irritated, which affects breathing. Demulcents have an anti-inflammatory and soothing effect on the kidneys, bladder, and mucous membranes. They also help moisten these tissues. Comfrey, licorice, marshmallow, and slippery elm are all demulcents.

Diaphoretics

Diaphoretics cause you to perspire, thus eliminating toxins through the skin. By dilating capillaries near the skin's surface, which also improves overall blood circulation, or relaxing pores, diaphoretics cause toxins to more easily pass into sweat glands, where they are discarded once you shower. Athletes who have problems sweating may benefit from such herbs. Diaphoretics also support the kidneys, where toxins are separated from the blood and discarded in the urine. Some herbs with a diaphoretic action include basil, chrysanthemum, ginger, lemon balm, and peppermint.

Diuretics

By increasing the production and removal of urine, diuretics also eliminate toxins and waste from the body. Ancient herbal tradition has it that diuretics include any herb beneficial to the urinary system's overall health. Many herbs, including parsley root, uva ursi, cornsilk, alfalfa, juniper berries, artichokes, asparagus, astragalus, buchu, burdock, celery, chaparral, dandelion, kava kava, and sarsaparilla, are known to have diuretic properties. Diuretics should not be used long-term and definitely not during intense exercise as they can rob you of several minerals, especially from your blood, and body fluids, both of which are vital during exercise.

Expectorants

Expectorants are commonly referred to as herbs that help the lungs. While they do indeed help your lungs, they do so by removing phlegm and excess fluid from them as well as the throat. Expectorants are also useful for bronchitis, pleurisy, and pneumonia. Such herbs include coltsfoot, elecampane, and mullein.

In addition to expectorants, other herbs can help optimize lung health. Mullein, besides being an expectorant, also serves as a lung tonic and anti-inflammatory. Other expectorant herbs include sundew, wild cherry bark, skunk cabbage, and bloodroot.

Hepatics

Hepatics aid liver function. The liver is an important organ for many reasons, including waste removal. Athletes experience ammonia toxicity resulting from the breakdown of protein for energy; the liver eliminates ammonia. Athletes suffer from a buildup of lactic acid resulting from the breakdown of glycogen during exercise; the liver eliminates lactic acid. Some ill-advised athletes resort to the use of illegal anabolic steroids, which are potentially harmful to the liver. You get the picture. Athletes definitely need a peak performing liver! Hepatics can help increase bile production and waste removal and detoxify the liver. Barberry, dandelion root, Oregon grapes, milk thistle, balmony, and gentian are some useful hepatics.

Hypotensives

Hypotensives help normalize blood pressure. Obviously, this is an important category for those who have high blood pressure. Hawthorn, linden blossoms, ginkgo biloba, garlic, and motherwort are all excellent hypotensives.

Hypnotics

Do not be misled by the term *hypnotic*; they will not put you into a trance, put you to sleep for hours, or cause you to hallucinate. Hypnotics gently help you fall asleep quicker and improve the quality of sleep. Proper sleep patterns are hard to come by for some. Traveling to games, the stress of performing well, the stress of balancing academics and athletics, and numerous other causes can keep you awake at night. Obviously, energy levels are negatively affected from lack of adequate sleep, but sleep also affects growth-hormone output and recovery from workouts and injuries.

Herbs such as valerian, California poppy, lobelia, skullcap, lemon balm, and peppermint can all calm you down for a night's rest!

Laxatives

Laxatives are a multimillion-dollar business for the pharmaceutical industry, but many herbs also serve as laxatives and are much gentler on the body, and less expensive, than commercial brands. Stimulating bowel movements removes wastes and toxins from the body, but body fluids and vital minerals are also lost. So, as with diuretics, caution should be used when taking laxative herbs. Do not prolong your use of laxatives. Some natural laxatives include cascara sagrada, dandelion root, psyllium seeds, senna leaf, aloe vera, boneset, and damiana.

Male and Female Reproductive Herbs

Proper functioning of your reproductive system will do far more for your athletic career than continue your legacy of athletic achievement! An array of health benefits can be gained by normalizing your hormonal balance. Take note: your hormonal balance is strongly affected by your reproductive system, and hormones affect all functions and systems of the body! Therefore, herbs that benefit the reproductive system can ease menopause, moodiness, and sexual dysfunction, as well as promote proper hormonal balance. This in turn may enhance tissue repair, improve liver function, provide more efficient digestion and assimilation, and amplify energy levels, metabolic functions, and brain activity.

Caution: when dealing with the hormonal balance of your body, great care should be taken. Even a slight change of this balance can cause an array of problems. Chasteberry, for example, contains phytochemicals that promote the balance of progesterone and estrogen, normally regarded as female hormones. It should not be taken by adolescent males but can be useful for females and older men.

Wild yams, black cohosh, saw palmetto, damiana, chasteberry, St. John's wort, oats, and those herbs with bitter properties have positive effects on the male reproductive system.

Chasteberry, blue cohosh, black cohosh, and bitter herbs have positive effects on the female reproductive system.

Nervines

Nervines have beneficial effects on the nervous system—the brain, central nervous system, neuromuscular system, as well as the sympathetic and parasympathetic nervous systems (those that bring impulses to and from your organs). Herbs that can help your nervous system include oats (the entire plant), skullcap, St. John's wort, motherwort, lobelia, and valerian.

Tonics

Tonics vitalize and nourish either one organ of the body or the entire body. The term *tonic* may bring visions of snake oils sold out of the back of covered wagons by peddlers traveling from town to town in the old West. While many such tonics may have been worthless, many weren't. Chances are people back in the old West were as eager for a quick solution to their ailments as they are today. Still, many herbs work remarkably well over time by gently coaxing your body back to good health or by aiding in maintaining health. Noted herbalist James Green had this to say about tonics:

> [Tonics are] perhaps the most important contribution herbal medicine can make in the process of natural healing. Tonic herbs stimulate nutrition by improving the assimilation of essential nutrients by the organs, improve systemic tone giving increased vigor, energy, and strength to the tissues of either specific organs or to the whole body. This is the central essential action to consider when devising any healing therapeutic formula. The other herbal actions work symbolically with toning to evolve relief and full healing.

Unlike chemical drugs of today, tonics help prevent health problems and can be taken with very little worry of side effects or overdose. While tonics should be used in times of good health, they can be especially helpful at the first signs of illness.

In fact, in each of the following chapters of this book, the first herbal preparation mentioned for each specific athletic goal is a tonic. We believe that the holistic approach to training and competition is best served this way. The following table lists the traditional tonics for each body system, while Appendix B lists the important tonics for athletes.

HERBAL TONICS AND THEIR SYSTEM AFFINITY

System	Herbal Tonics
Liver and bile	goldenseal, Oregon grape root, dandelion root, fennel
Blood	dong quai, lycii berries, rehmannia
Heart	hawthorn, motherwort
Energy	astragalus, ginseng, jujube dates, licorice
Immune system	reishi, astragalus, schizandra
Nervous system	skullcap, valerian
Sexual functions	dong quai, ginseng, licorice
Digestive system	codonopsis, elecampane
Urinary system	parsley, rehmannia
Overall nutrient	comfrey, marshmallow, slippery elm
Lung	mullein

SUMMARY OF PHYSIOLOGICAL ACTIONS OF HERBS

Classification	Action	Useful Herbs
Adaptogens	regulate stress	Siberian ginseng, chaparral, dandelion root, aloe vera, echinacea, yellow dock, goldenseal
Alteratives	normalize bodily functions	Nettle, cleavers, burdock, dandelion, yellow dock, red clover, chaparral, Oregon grapes
Anticatarrhals	rid body of excess mucous	goldenrod, elder tree, eyebright
Anti-inflammatories	reduce swelling of tissues	chamomile, lemon balm, peppermint, meadowsweet, willow bark, bog bean, wild yams
Antimicrobials and antibacterials	fight micro-organisms and harmful bacteria	chaparral, echinacea, garlic, goldenseal
Antispasmodics	relieve muscle cramping and tension	black haw, grindelia, lobelia, angelica, peppermint
Astringents	bond and firm tissues	white oak, pipsissewa, horse chestnut, witch hazel, agrimony, cranesbill
Bitters	detoxify	gentian, citrus peel, angelica, barberry, burdock, dandelion, mugwort, horehound, elecampane, turmeric, ginseng
Calmatives and Carminatives	improve digestive system	fennel, rosemary, cumin, ginger, peppermint

SUMMARY OF PHYSIOLOGICAL ACTIONS OF HERBS (*continued*)

Classification	Action	Useful Herbs
Demulcents	improve kidney and urinary system health; promote moistening of mucous membranes	comfrey, licorice, marshmallow, slippery elm
Diaphoretics	eliminate toxins via perspiration	basil, chrysanthemum, ginger, lemon balm, peppermint
Diuretics	eliminate toxins and waste via urinary system	parsley root, uva ursi, cornsilk, alfalfa, juniper berries, artichokes, asparagus, astragalus, buchu, burdock, celery, chaparral, dandelion, kava kava, sarsaparilla
Reproductive system	normalize hormonal balance; normalize reproductive system	Male: wild yams, black cohosh, saw palmetto, damiana, chasteberry, St. John's wort, wild oats, bitter herbs Female: chasteberry, blue cohosh, black cohosh, bitter herbs
Hepatics	aid in liver functions	barberry, dandelion root, Oregon grapes, milk thistle, balmony, gentian
Hypotensives	regulate blood pressure	hawthorn, linden blossoms, ginkgo biloba, garlic, motherwort
Hypnotics	improve quality of sleep	valerian, California poppy, lobelia, skullcap, lemon balm, peppermint, Siberian ginseng

SUMMARY OF PHYSIOLOGICAL ACTIONS OF HERBS *(continued)*

Classification	Action	Useful Herbs
Laxatives	eliminate wastes via bowel movements	cascara sagrada, dandelion root, psyllium seeds, aloe vera, boneset, damiana
Expectorants	remove excess fluid from lungs and throat; promote lung vitality	mullein, sundew, wild cherry bark, skunk cabbage, bloodroot
Hepatics	detoxify the liver; promote liver vitality	barberry, dandelion root, Oregon grapes, gentian
Nervines	promote nervous system health	oats, skullcap, St. John's wort, motherwort, lobelia, valerian
Rubefacients	stimulate blood flow to the skin	black pepper, cayenne, mustard
Tonics	promote overall vitality of organs and systems	goldenseal, Oregon grapes, dandelion root, fennel, dong quai, lycii berries, rehmannia, hawthorn, motherwort, astragalus, jujube dates, licorice, reishi, schizandra, skullcap, valerian, codonopsis, elecampane, parsley, comfrey, marshmallow, slippery elm
Vulneraries	promote healing of cuts, bruises, tissue irritation, inflammation	arcica, calendula, chickweed

Some herbs listed in the preceding table may cause unwanted symptoms to appear or be illegal in sports competition. We strongly recommend that you read the disclaimer at the beginning of this book and consult with an herbalist skilled in both sports training and sports medicine before using any of these herbs.

Rubefacients

Rubefacients stimulate blood flow near the skin when applied topically. Because of this action, rubefacients are useful for most athletes because they promote healing and reduce the symptoms of arthritis, joint, and muscle pain. Black pepper, cayenne, mustard, and mint family herbs are listed among the many known rubefacients.

Vulneraries

Vulneraries are a category of herbs those involved in contact sports will definitely want to check out. Vulneraries promote healing of cuts, abrasions, and bruises; relieve tissue irritations; and promote blood flow to areas affected by bruises and inflamed tissues. Arnica, calendula, and chickweed are known vulneraries.

Methods of Preparing Herbs

We do *not* expect you to prepare your own herbal supplements. You cannot simply run out to the woods or fields and gather the appropriate foliage, roots, berries, flowers, barks, or seeds and consume them. In Appendix C we have listed the manufacturers with whom we have dealt over the years and know to be excellent sources for prepared herbs. Preparing herbs yourself is fraught with difficulties you may not expect. Here are four good reasons for going to the health food store or herbalist:

1. You may have to eat massive quantities of the herb to get the desired result.
2. Some plants can be unhealthy or even dangerous.
3. Some herbs can taste downright horrible.
4. The right part of the plant has to be prepared.

Because of these factors, herbal supplement manufacturers and herbalists have developed ways to prepare herbs so that potency, safety, effectiveness, and palatability are enhanced.

Soaking herbs in hot liquid to make a tea is known as *infusion*. In this case the herb obviously has to taste good, and the heat cannot make any of the active phytochemicals stronger or weaker. The hot water provides a soothing delivery system as well as a means of dissolving or releasing the active compounds of the plant.

The process of *decoction* is used to separate the most important nutrients of an herb from unnecessary parts. This is the preferred method when using bark, roots, seeds, or other parts of plants you wouldn't want on your dinner plate.

Many herbs are ground into a *powder* and placed in a capsule. In fact, most herbs can be prepared and purchased in this fashion. The benefits of encapsulating herbs is obvious: you won't have to taste an herb you don't particularly care for, and measurements can be made in a precise manner.

Tinctures are made by grinding an herb or combination of herbs into a powder and mixing the powder with water and alcohol. This is a very popular method for herb usage because it is a cost-effective way to store herbs for a long period of time.

Extracts are made by boiling herbs down to a thick, super-concentrated syrup, and then mixing it with alcohol. Extracts can be four to eight times more concentrated than tinctures.

Herbs can also be used as *ointments*, hydrotherapeutic *baths*, and *fomentations* (soaking a cloth in a decoction) for external application. These applications are useful for bruises, swellings, cuts, and burns.

Proper Use and Dosage of Herbs

As we pointed out in the previous section, it is unlikely that you will ever overdose on herbs that you purchase in a health food store or from an herbalist because herbal supplements are almost always manufactured following standardized dosages. In fact, it is more likely that you will take too little of the herb than too much. Manufacturers often recommend conservative dosages. For example, the dosage of most capsules used by herbal supplement manufacturers is approximately 750–800 milligrams, which is the size most people can swallow comfortably. However, since the optimal dose of many commonly used herbs is 2–4 grams (2,000–4,000 milligrams), you would be required to swallow up to five or six of these capsules at a time. Since this can be both uncomfortable to some people as well as expensive, not to mention a "tough sell" from a marketing point of view, the manufacturer may decide to recommend two capsules daily. Assuming that money isn't a problem, the logical way around the problem of lower-than-optimal dosage recommendation would be to take one or two capsules before each of your three-to-five daily meals.

If you have any questions pertaining to dosage and side effects, and you cannot find the pertinent information in this text or elsewhere, we urge you to seek the advice of an herbalist skilled in the sports medical and sports conditioning sciences. Following are a few general guidelines on how herbal dosages are typically established:

- Many herbs, particularly adaptogens that are actually consumed as foods, often have dosages of 2 to 4 grams (or 2 to 4 milliliters of tincture) three times daily. With such herbs, it is not critical to be exact.
- When the instructions on the herb packaging advise a recommended dosage of 1 to 2 grams or less, care is generally advised, since the herb may be potent or accompanied by some uncomfortable side effects. But there's usually no need for paranoia.
- Potentially dangerous or highly concentrated herbs are rarely found in health food stores, as manufacturers are wary of selling them. In fact, the FDA has restricted the sale and distribution of almost all of the more dangerous medicinal herbs, even to herbalists. Nonetheless, when the recommended dosage is under 1 gram or 1 milliliter, it generally signifies that far greater care must be taken in their use.
- Herbalists traditionally recommend a full (maximum recommended) dose of an herb that targets the most important organ or symptom of an illness or injury, and a lesser dose of those herbs whose actions are secondary to the main problem.
- Children are generally given herbal tonics for their special needs both because they are relatively safe and because the

self-healing power of children is exceptionally high. We do *not* recommend that you treat youngsters as grown athletes, and because of this, we do *not* recommend the same herbs for them that we recommend for adults. Having said this, we nonetheless feel that you should be aware of the relationship between age (body weight) and dosages of the more common herbs, established by the British National Formulary in 1985:

Age	Body Weight (lb.)	Percent of adult dose
Newborn	7.5	12.5
1 month	9	14.5
3 months	12	18
6 months	17	22
1 year	22	25
3 years	31	33
7 years	51	50
12 years	81	75
Adult male	150	100
Adult female	123	100

The table beginning on the next page lists some of the herbs that you should only use under a sports herbalist's expert supervision or avoid altogether.

HERBS CONSIDERED UNSAFE OR UNFIT FOR HUMAN USE

Common name	Source	Use	Safety/Efficacy/Dosage
Borage	*Borago officinalis* Leaves and tops	diuretic, antidiarrheal	Both safety and efficacy are questionable; contains toxic pyrrolizidine alkaloids, including intermedine, lycopsamine, amabiline, and supinine.
Calamus	*Acorus calamus*	febrifuge, digestive aid rhizome (underground stem)	Chemovars (plants that have similar appearances but have different chemical compositions) contain varying amounts of carcinogenic cisisonsarone. Indian type most toxic; North American type is nontoxic; test for cisisonasarone before using.
Chaparral	*Larrea tridentata* leaves and twigs	anticancer	Currently not recommended—no proven efficacy; purported to induce severe liver toxicity, but limited number of cases have been seen, in spite of widespread use. Further investigation required.
Coltsfood	*Tussilago farfara* leaves	antitiussive, demulcent	Effective but unsafe; contains carcinogenic pyrrolizidine alkaloids including senkirkine and senecionine.
Comfrey	*Symphytum* species rhizome and roots, leaves	wound healing	Effective but unsafe for internal use; contains large number of toxic pyrrolizidine alkaloids, which vary according to species.

HERBS CONSIDERED UNSAFE OR UNFIT FOR HUMAN USE (*continued*)

Common name	Source	Use	Safety/Efficacy/Dosage
Ephedra (Ma huang)	*Ephedra sinica* and related species green stems	anorectic, bronchodilator	Relatively ineffective as an anorectic; effective for bronchodilation; unsafe for those suffering from hypertension, diabetes, or thyroid disease. Avoid consumption with caffeine.
Germander	*Teucrium chamaedrys* leaves and tops	anorectic	Unsafe and ineffective; causes hepatotoxicity because of diterpernoid derivatives.
Life root	*Senecio aureus* whole plant	emmenagogue	Unsafe (hepatotoxic) and no proven efficacy; contains toxic pyrrolizidine alkaloids.
Pokeroot	*Phytolacca americana*	alterative (tonic), antirheumatic, anticancer	Unsafe and ineffective; should not be sold or used. May be fatal to children.
Sassafras	*Sassafras albidum* root bark	stimulant, antispasmodic, antirheumatic, tonic	Unsafe and ineffective; volatile oil contains carcinogenic safrole.

Source: Donald R. Counts, M.D. (http://www.drcounts.com/convmed.html)

In their zeal to excel, athletes often "shotgun" several supplements daily. This can lead to problems if one or two of the more
potent herbs are repeated in several of the different supplements.
We recommend that you always read the label carefully when you
purchase herbal supplements. Then you will be able to carefully
monitor the amount of each herb being used.

In summary, while a great majority of the herbs recommended in
this book (and others that are readily available in health food stores
everywhere) are generally regarded as safe, it is always advisable to
take the following precautions:

- Read the labels on all supplements being used, and know the
  total amount of each herb you're taking.
- Seek competent assistance from a qualified sports herbalist,
  particularly with more potent herbs.
- Remember that many herbs are banned from use in sports by
  most of the sports governing bodies of the world, including the
  International Olympic Committee. So always read the rules of
  your sport and check with your team physician *before* getting
  into trouble. The use of these herbs is considered "doping."
- Do not give powerful herbs to children—opt instead for mild
  tinctures. If you have any questions whatsoever (and there
  almost always should be questions), you should seek advice
  from a pediatrician.
- If you are on any medication whatsoever, it is quite likely that
  some of the phytochemicals in your herbal supplements may
  cause unwanted interactions. Always check with your physician
  and sports herbalist before you use herbs while medicated.

3

Training and Nutrition for Peak Performance

Asking the question "Why do athletes train?" seems a silly thing to do. "To get better at their sport!" would be the standard reply. However, ask the question anyway. Look deeper for answers. Here are a few you'll come up with:

- To get stronger
- To get bigger muscles
- To reduce body fat
- For better anaerobic energy
- For better aerobic energy
- For better mental focus, arousal, or concentration
- To reduce pain
- To speed wound healing
- To improve between-workout recovery
- For general systemic health

There is a broad array of technologies available to help modern athletes improve the chances of accomplishing these training objectives. The application of any one of them has an effect on all the others. What you eat affects how you run. How and when you run affects your weight training, which in turn affects how you eat, your mental state, your overall health, and your skill. All affect each other in

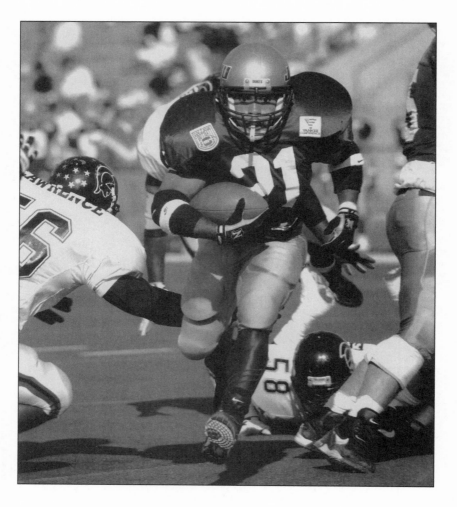

Ever see a hole this big before? Things like this do not merely "happen" in sports. They come from perfect preparation and execution. Everything you do in training takes on monumental importance when you focus on peak performance. It is the same in life. How you manipulate your training, caloric intake, supplementation, and all other facets of your sports preparation will be reflected in how you think, feel, and play the game.

myriad ways—most predictable and, therefore, controllable. This is the art and science of modern sports conditioning.

These are the eight training technologies used by contemporary athletes:

1. weight training (barbells, dumbbells, weight machines)
2. special forms of training (calisthenics, running, plyometrics, stretching)
3. psychological techniques and strategies (self-hypnosis, mental imagery, transcendental meditation)
4. various therapeutic modalities (whirlpool, massage, infrared irradiation, electrical stimulation)
5. medical support (regular checkups, drug therapy, chiropractic adjustments)
6. biomechanical and motor learning systems (skill training)
7. dietary manipulation techniques (what, how, and when to eat to accomplish specific sports-related objectives)
8. herbs and other supplements (ergogenic aids)

The Integrated Approach To Training

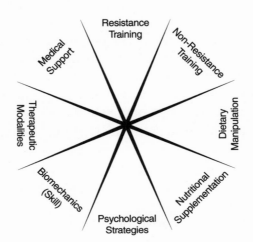

The spokes of the wheel represent each of the eight training technologies. It is clear that with all spokes intact, the wheel is made stronger. So, too, will be your sports-performance efforts. With each missing spoke, your performance deteriorates until you simply cannot endure the rigors of sports training or competition.

Herbs are an important part of this picture and have the ability to make your training more efficient. Herbs can aid in improving your mental focus and sharpening your senses. Some herbs are used to improve recovery, aid in healing, and make you run faster or lift heavier weights. The point is that by knowing about the power of herbs, you can make appropriate adjustments to your training regimen so that the benefits of herbs are available to you.

However, you will not reap the maximum benefits of herbs unless you know how to manipulate your training and how and when to apply each training technology. One simple example illustrates how this is done. If you recover faster, you are able to work out more frequently. But if you don't work out more frequently, what value is there in speeding recovery? None. So it behooves you to understand what sports conditioning entails before you can adequately benefit from the use of herbs or any other technology.

Performance Nutrition

The word *food* is generally restricted to the things we eat that contain macronutrients (protein, carbohydrates, and fat) and micronutrients (vitamins, minerals, and trace elements). However, make no mistake about it, many of the plants we eat as food sources also contain phytochemicals that are helpful in many ways. Further, macronutrients and micronutrients found in many food sources also have potent druglike action in our bodies because they exert a profound influence on the powerful hormones and enzymes that we need to survive, grow, and perform optimally. One such druglike action is of central concern in this chapter. That is, how the food we eat controls insulin. In fact, food is the only thing that can control insulin. So, we need to understand the elemental qualities of a performance-nutrition protocol.

Animals eat to survive. Some have adapted to their environment rather well and have learned to eat grass or other plants that force them to regurgitate any spoiled food they consume. That's part of survival. And humans, like animals, have also learned to eat things that'll help them survive. But humans learned long ago to eat for reasons beyond mere energy and growth requirements. They learned to eat for pleasure and for health and healing, and herbs are among those things humans learned to eat. Paradoxically, humans have also taken on the curious habit of putting things in their bodies that can kill them or make them ill. A widely contaminated public water supply, booze, cigarettes, cocaine, pesticides, and additives—you name it! Just the mere thought of some of these poisons can make you sick!

Rules of Performance Nutrition

Unlike normal folks, athletes have learned to eat for many reasons beyond survival, health, and pleasure. Athletes are focused on performance, so their eating habits reflect this all-consuming passion. In the remainder of this book, we will delve deeper into how athletes eat. First, though, here are some rules all should follow when designing a performance diet:

Rule One: Always eat at least five times a day. Two or three meals simply aren't often enough. It's permissible to regard two of these meals as snacks, provided they are comprised of sufficient calories to get you to your next meal, and they are comprised of the appropriate ratio of macronutrients as described in Rules Two and Three. By eating more frequently, you will control your blood sugar and insulin levels (and thus your energy level), you'll get protein in small amounts throughout the day to support growth and recovery, and most important, body fat will be mobilized as an energy source rather than stored. Simply, by providing your body with a consistent and frequent supply of just the right number of calories, you significantly reduce its need to store fat. Conversely, when you eat infrequently, your body recognizes a "famine" situation, and your entire endocrine system (powerful hormones produced inside your body that control how you grow, recover, and produce energy) is thrown for a loop. Then too much of the food you consume is stored as body fat in preparation for the famine to come.

Rule Two: In planning each of your daily meals or snacks, begin with a ratio of approximately one part fat, two parts protein, and three parts carbohydrates. However, as you will see in Rule Three, this is merely an estimate for average people. Depending on the severity of your daily work routine and training protocol, you may need more or fewer carbohydrates for energy. Fat is essential for maintaining good health, and it is needed to manufacture many important hormones in your body, so *do not* attempt to eliminate fats from your diet! Just try to ensure that saturated fat from animal sources is kept low and unsaturated fats such as canola oil or olive oil predominate. Also, you must consume enough protein to support growth and recovery and enough carbohydrates (primarily low-glycemic-index carbohydrates that are converted to blood sugar slowly—the best food sources are nontropical fruits and beans of all varieties) to control your insulin levels. Remember, carbohydrates are your body's preferred energy fuel source, although fats work well, too, particularly during aerobic training—provided the ratio of fats, protein, and carbohydrates is kept within the recommended levels. Remember that protein and carbohydrates both have four calories per gram, while fat has nine calories per gram.

Rule Three: When you sit down to eat, ask yourself, "What am I going to be doing for the next three hours of my life?" Then, if you're taking a nap, eat fewer carbohydrates; if you're planning a training session, eat more carbohydrates. And so forth. In other words, your carbs are adjusted up or down depending on anticipated energy output. Remember, though, that your pre-workout carbohydrates must be of the variety that convert to blood sugar slowly.

Rule Four: You can't lose fat quickly and efficiently unless you're on a negative-calorie diet—taking in fewer calories than you would need to stay the same weight. Neither can you gain muscle tissue quickly and efficiently unless you're on a positive-calorie diet—taking in more calories than you'd need to maintain your current weight. So, how can you gain muscle and lose fat at the same time? Clearly, you can't. So you must alternate periods of negative-calorie balance with periods of positive-calorie balance. It doesn't matter if you're trying to lose total body weight, stay at the same total body weight, or gain total body weight. Alternating in this way will (1) readjust your basal metabolic rate (BMR) upward, making it easier to keep the fat off, and (2) control your body's hormones, especially your insulin and glucagon. (Glucagon is a hormone that stimulates the breakdown of sugar stored in muscles—glycogen—as well as in the liver—glucose—and gives you greater energy.) You support recovery and lean tissue building and at the same time retard fat deposition. Remember, if you want to put on lean muscle at the same time you're taking off fat, you *must* zigzag your calories! So, depending on your goal, follow one of these guidelines:

- *To increase total body weight by losing fat and gaining muscle:* For four to five days each week (including training days), add two calories per pound of lean body weight to your normal daily caloric intake according to the rules we've discussed. Spread these added calories among five meals per day. For example, a 170-pound person who is around 12 percent body fat should add approximately 300 calories per day. Over five meals, that equals about 60 calories per meal. Then on the remaining two to three days each week (including off days or light training days), reduce your caloric intake by two calories per pound of lean body weight. Reduce each of your five meals per day according to rules. For example, a 170-pound person who is around 12 percent body fat should subtract approximately 300 calories per day. Over five meals, that equals a 60-calorie decrease per meal on average. Don't forget to adjust your calories upward each month to reflect the new caloric needs of your increased muscle mass.
- *To decrease total body weight by losing fat and gaining muscle:* For four to five days each week (especially on off days and light training days), reduce your caloric intake by two calories per pound of lean body weight as previously described. Then on the remaining two to three days each week (including heavy training days), add two calories per pound of lean body weight to your normal daily caloric intake. Don't forget to adjust your calories upward each month to reflect the new caloric needs of your increased muscle mass.
- *To stay the same total body weight but lose fat and gain muscle:* For three to four days each week (especially on off days or light training days) reduce your caloric intake by two calories per pound of lean body weight. Increase your caloric intake for the other three or four days each week (especially on heavy training days) by two calories per pound of lean body weight. Don't forget to adjust your calories upward each month to reflect the new caloric needs of your increased muscle mass.

Rule Five: It is almost impossible to get all the nutrients your body needs to remain healthy and active from food alone, particularly if you're in your negative-calorie period. So, it's important to supplement your diet with vitamins, minerals, and other carefully selected substances to ensure maximum progress toward your fitness, health, muscle-building, and fat-loss goals. Also, no matter how hard you try, no matter how good a cook you are, or where you buy your food:

- You can't always eat five or six times daily.
- There are many instances in which your body either requires or can make good use of certain micronutrients in greater amounts than can be derived from food alone.
- A perfectly balanced diet cannot be maintained during periods of contest preparation or periods where there is a purposeful caloric restriction imposed.
- Soil depletion, toxins in the food chain, overprocessing, overcooking, free-radical formation in the body, and a host of other sometimes medically related factors all interact to make food less than totally nutritious or adequate in providing sound health and optimal fitness.
- Periods of high-stress training require supernormal intake of many nutrients without a commensurate increase in caloric needs.
- Periods of high-stress training create a situation in which various benefits can be derived from substances not normally found in food or biosynthesized in the body in sufficient quantities, but which are easily derived from botanical sources.
- Human genius has improved on Mother Nature's original work in many of life's arenas. One such arena is in the nutritional supplement industry. There are some great supplements to one's diet for serious sports competition training or fitness training that are not available in nature as a food source or an herbal preparation.

So, you must use both herbs and nutritional supplements!

Any other rules would certainly include (1) drinking plenty of clean, filtered water throughout the day, and (2) abstaining from herbal or man-made drugs, smoking, and overuse of alcohol. In addition to being unhealthy, and in many instances against the law, such substances limit your ability to achieve your sports or fitness goals.

These five rules must literally direct your athletic life! Following them can mean the difference between winning and losing, between peak performance and good performance, between star status and a second-place finish. Athletes strive to excel, and this must begin with scientific eating habits. Let's look at some reasons athletes should pay close attention to how they eat.

Stronger, Bigger Muscles

You can either stay the same weight you are now, lose weight, or gain weight. In all three cases you'll want to put on muscle and take off fat. In the world of sports where strength-to-weight ratio means everything, there is no other way! You have three choices: You can (1) stay the same total weight but increase your lean mass, (2) gain total body weight by adding muscle, or (3) reduce your total body weight but get more muscle. Re-read Rule Four to get a clear handle on this process.

Better Anaerobic and Aerobic Energy

There is a high degree of specificity in the energy output required of athletes in a host of different sports. This demands careful nutritional support. It is important to realize that not all athletes react the same to food consumption during training or competition. You must know how your body reacts to various foods before you reach competition. Here are some factors to consider when you're matching your nutrition to your training needs:

Explosive athletes—those who complete their skill or event in a few seconds—only use ATP (adenosine triphosphate) and CP (creatine phosphate) for producing the energy they need. ATP molecules are split apart, giving energy for muscle contraction; CP is then split apart to replenish diminishing ATP. They should attempt to stimulate the storage of glycogen in muscles while promoting repair and growth of muscle tissue and inhibiting fat deposits. This can be done by following these suggestions:

- Train anaerobically (to exhaustion) on a regular basis. Through intense training you stimulate increased storage of muscle and liver glycogen. This permits additional levels of energy for greater work loads.
- Follow the five rules of nutrition described above.
- Consume adequate amounts of water. Not only does consuming adequate water reduce your chances of dehydration, but for every gram of glycogen stored within your muscle, three grams of water is stored along with it. And being dehydrated can weaken muscle contractions and bring on fatigue.

Mid-distance athletes—those whose skill or event requires force output for several seconds up to five minutes or so—must break down stored sugar inside their muscles to produce the energy they need. Here are a few pointers on providing nutrition for the stamina needed to compete in middle-distance events:

- Train against the anaerobic threshold on a regular basis.
- Follow the five rules of performance nutrition described above.
- Consume adequate amounts of water.

Long-distance or endurance athletes must deliver large quantities of oxygen to their working muscles and to their heart in order to produce the energy they need. The source of energy used during aerobic exercise depends on the duration and intensity of activity. For instance, within 1½ to two hours of endurance training, the glycogen content of the muscles and liver can become depleted. At this time, athletes might experience what is known as "hitting the wall."

Although it is somewhat easy to deplete carbohydrate stores it is quite impossible to deplete fat stores. But fat cannot be used as energy unless some carbohydrates are present in the muscle cells and liver. Therefore, it is not likely that an endurance athlete can rely on fat for energy when glycogen stores are completely drained. So, you must consume a diet that allows you to spare glycogen use, so fat can be used as a main source of fuel. This can be accomplished by adhering to the following practices:

- Regularly train for endurance. By participating in long-term aerobic activity, you will be capable of storing two times the amount of glycogen as an inactive person. You will also have the capability of storing one and half times more intramuscular fat as an inactive person. This permits more carbohydrate-based fuel to be available to your working muscles along with increased fat burning for energy.

- Follow the five rules of performance nutrition described above.
- Do not fat-load. Fat-loading was thought to be of benefit to endurance athletes in order to promote fat-based energy. But problems persist with this practice—for example, you will be faced with increased urination which can cause loss of minerals essential to healthy heart action.
- Do not consume carbohydrates one and half to two hours before an endurance activity. The ingestion of carbohydrates reduces your chances of mobilizing and using free fatty acids as energy. Your body will use glycogen stores for energy, forcing you to fatigue sooner.
- Consume carbohydrates during aerobic activities. Because exercise lowers the release of insulin into your bloodstream, the consumption of carbohydrates spares glycogen use and allows fat to be used for energy. Carbohydrate drinks with a low glycemic index will provide you with sustained blood sugar levels, preserving glycogen stores.
- Drink plenty of water. Endurance athletes sweat profusely, losing valuable fluids and minerals. By consuming water throughout your training and during competition, you can help prevent dehydration that can reduce your performance and be potentially dangerous to your health. To protect against deficiencies in any nutrients, a multi-vitamin and mineral supplement is suggested. During endurance activity, you should drink four to six ounces of fluid every 15 to 30 minutes. For every pound you lose from sweating you should consume one pint of fluid. And chilled fluids absorb faster.

Better Mental Focus, Arousal, or Concentration

By far the best method of maintaining or improving your concentration abilities is to eat properly. The previous section on energy needs applies here. However, certain other factors can be considered in improving these important elements of peak performance.

For example, adequate sleep is clearly conducive to alertness throughout the day. And there are several techniques for improving clarity of thought and eliminating unwanted "mental noise" during training or competition. These techniques may include therapeutic modalities of various sorts, herbs, transcendental meditation, visualization training, stress-reduction strategies, pain-reduction strategies, and many others. These are covered in detail in Chapter 10.

Improved Between-Workout Recovery

Failure to adapt in sports results in injury. Bruises and wounds of various sorts are omnipresent in sports and must be treated if peak performance ability is to be had. Once treated, you would hope some sort of adaptive mechanism would prevent a recurrence and allow progress to continue. It doesn't always work that way, so get used to it! In Chapter 7, we'll explore some herbal as well as nonherbal adaptogens. We'll also look at some interesting herbal and nonherbal restorative agents. Then we'll explore how your immune system works, what you can do to boost your immune competence— and what that will mean for improved sports performance. Finally, various lifestyle factors, once harnessed, can work for you instead of against you.

General Systemic Health

To an athlete, "Pay me now or pay me later" means, "You can try to stay healthy, or get sick and then try to get better." You know, like preventive maintenance on your car will save money in the long run. So true for your body as well!

Holistic theory tells us that balance and harmony are the keys to prevention. And, make no mistake about it, your body is only part of the story of prevention. There must be clear and free flow of energy through the various aspects of your life besides the physical. So, there is a range of issues that go beyond transforming metabolic and physiological processes that must be addressed:

- Nutrition must be of a quality that ensures both health and peak performance ability.

- Physiological and structural factors involving overall physical fitness must somehow merge with sports excellence. Remember this: there is no such thing as a "fit" athlete! Why? Because you must totally focus on those physical attributes which will allow you to perform optimally. That sometimes means you must purposefully disregard other elements of overall physical fitness. Still, in the off-season, you have to go back to basics and re-establish a base of overall fitness.
- Your emotional life is fundamental to achieving peak performance capabilities as well as sound health. No, you needn't solicit the services of a psychotherapist or anything that radical. But certainly being aware of your emotional needs is critical to your overall health.
- The Bible says that without vision the people die. Without a personal vision, life becomes a slow process of degeneration and decay. So, good health depends in large part on some form of critical thought being given to who you really are, who you want to become, and how you're going to get there.
- Spirituality is vital to maintaining overall health. To most, the word *spirituality* relates to how closely you believe in and follow the precepts of a particular religion. On the other hand, it can also involve an appreciation for beauty, susceptibility to the inner joy offered in poetry or art, or nothing more than finding joy in being alive.

Consuming energizing calories before workouts and competition is important. But peak performance can only be achieved if you consume the right amount. Too much or too little carbohydrate-rich food can hinder performance. Use the following chart to establish your specific needs.

ACTIVITIES AND THEIR APPROXIMATE HOURLY CALORIC COST FOR VARIOUS BODY WEIGHTS

If you weigh . . .	125	150	175	200	225	250	275	300
Light aerobics	154	204	254	304	354	404	454	504
Walking 2.5 MPH	154	204	204	304	354	404	454	504
Gardening	168	218	268	318	368	418	468	518
Golf	195	245	295	345	395	445	505	545
Lawn mowing	195	245	295	345	395	445	505	545
Light calisthenics	222	272	322	372	422	472	522	572
Light weight training	222	272	322	372	422	472	522	572
Housecleaning	222	272	322	372	422	472	522	572
Walking 3.75 MPH	249	299	349	399	449	499	549	599
Swimming .25 MPH	249	299	349	399	449	499	549	599
Medium aerobics	290	340	390	440	490	540	590	640
Badminton	297	347	397	447	497	547	597	647
Wood chopping	344	394	444	494	544	594	644	694
Medium weight training	392	442	492	542	592	642	692	742
Slow jogging	426	476	526	576	626	676	726	776
Heavy calisthenics	494	544	594	644	694	744	794	844
Heavy aerobics	494	544	594	644	694	744	794	844
Heavy weight training	562	612	662	712	762	812	862	912
Cycling 13 MPH	610	660	710	760	810	860	910	960
Fast jogging	630	680	730	780	830	880	910	960

It is not an accident that the reasons athletes train and eat are coincident. In the remaining chapters of this book, we will discuss in greater depth the reasons athletes eat as they do, including herbal approaches for augmenting each. You will clearly see that, for those seeking peak performance ability, nutritional eating, supplementing, and training are inseparable disciplines.

4

Digestion and Assimilation of Foods

Not everyone is blessed with the genetic gift of being able to easily stimulate muscular growth. And given today's abusive diet of processed foods, chemical additives, alcohol, carbonated sugar drinks, and tobacco, it is easy to see why gastric upset, constipation, indigestion, and a host of other alimentary problems plague modern man.

The diet problem is easily solved by practicing abstention or moderation. As for genetics, sometimes Mother Nature can help nudge your system to get past a muscle-growth plateau. One way is to improve the efficiency of your digestive processes. Your digestive system is responsible for breaking food down into its component nutrients and then getting those nutrients into your bloodstream and on route to your cells. This digestive and assimilation process is an enormous task which takes several hours to complete. Not all of your food is fully digested; some is passed out of the body as waste.

Practicing both optimal nutrition and avoiding of the common toxins mentioned above are important parts of your integrated training. They are elemental to your ultimate success as an elite athlete. In fact, we believe that they are elemental to peak performance in general, whether you're a business executive, homemaker, or truck driver. We do not intend to chide you for your bad habits and inability or unwillingness to avoid or limit toxins. It is enough for you to

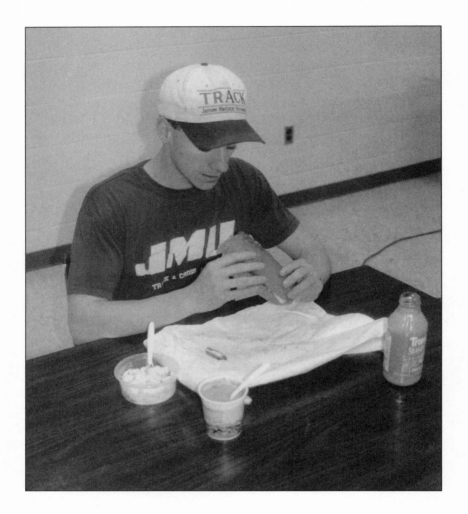

Many factors can impede or significantly reduce digestion and assimilation of food. This will invariably reduce recovery ability, energy levels, muscle growth, and general health.

know that it's important to do so. But, we can certainly show you a trick or two!

The digestive process can be improved. When it is improved, and when you follow the five steps of proper nutrition outlined in the last chapter, you will have more energy and be better able to optimize the muscle growth, recovery, and repair processes.

Your Digestive System

Your digestive process begins immediately upon putting food in your mouth. The food is broken down into tiny bits and mixed with your saliva, which contains some digestive enzymes. The bolus of food you swallow enters your stomach via your esophagus. When macronutrients—carbohydrates, protein, and fats—are eaten alone, they can pass through the stomach at a slightly faster rate. Carbohydrates are quickly passed, followed by protein, with fats taking the longest time. When these three macronutrients are consumed at the same time, as they usually are, it takes longer for them to be broken down and passed into your small intestine.

Your small intestine is called "small" because its diameter is much smaller than that of your large intestine. In fact, your small intestine is approximately twelve feet long and has much more mass than your large intestine. The major part of digestion occurs in the upper quadrant of your small intestine. This is where all nutrients, including protein, carbohydrates, fat, vitamins, minerals, and many of the herbs and other ergogenic supplements you take, are digested and absorbed into your bloodstream.

Undigested foods, especially indigestible fiber, pass through your small intestine into your large intestine. Your large intestine has two important jobs: (1) to absorb any water and electrolytes which may have passed through the small intestine, and (2) to move waste products to your bowels for removal.

Three more organs are involved in the digestion of your food: the liver, gallbladder, and pancreas. Your liver aids the digestive process by producing bile, a fluid containing salts, bile pigments, cholesterol, and other substances which are important for digestion. Your liver also plays an important role in metabolizing your carbohydrates and fats, and in the synthesis of protein. Your gallbladder stores excess bile. Your pancreas plays its role in digestion by producing pancreatic juice, a fluid which contains hormones and enzymes important in digesting starches, protein, and fat.

Digestion and Absorption of Carbohydrates

Carbohydrate digestion begins in your mouth where salivary amylase breaks some of the chemical binds which hold carbohydrates together. Unfortunately, most people don't chew their food long enough for this enzyme to take full effect. Starch, the most frequent carbohydrate you consume, is quite long in molecular structure and needs to be broken down into three separate molecules—short oligosaccharides, maltriose, and maltose—before it reaches the stomach. A small, but significant way to improve carbohydrate digestion is to make sure you chew your food long enough before shoving more food in!

Once these three molecules enter your small intestine, they are further broken down into monosaccharides which are easily absorbed into the bloodstream. If they arrive intact in the starch form, they must be broken down by a much slower process, which will slow absorption of all nutrients.

Glucose, a simple carbohydrate, can be partially absorbed in your stomach. For this reason, some sports drinks can be beneficial if taken no more than a half hour before intense physical activity, which will spare your body's glycogen stores to a degree. This technique is not advisable unless you are practicing, competing, or training, as it causes a rapid rise in your blood sugar level. This, in turn, causes an insulin response which leads to hypoglycemia and an attendant decrease in energy for quite some time.

Digestion and Absorption of Proteins

Protein digestion begins in your stomach when pepsin begins to break down long amino acid chains into shorter polypeptides. Further breakdown of these polypeptides occurs in your small intestine where several enzymes dismantle them in stepwise fashion until only free-form amino acids are left. Only then are they small enough to enter through the intestinal wall into the portal bloodstream.

Digestion and Absorption of Fats

Fat digestion does not begin until the fat reaches your small intestine. There, the fat is mixed with bile and pancreatic lipase. The fat is broken down into free fatty acids and monoglycerides and then passed through the intestinal wall. These fatty-acid and monoglyceride molecules are reassembled into triglycerides before entering the bloodstream.

Digestion and Absorption of Vitamins, Minerals, and Other Nutrients

Most of these micronutrients are absorbed in your small and large intestines, but some can be absorbed through the skin and mucous membranes of your mouth. Garlic is an excellent example. Even when you are chopping garlic, it is being absorbed through your fingertips. Most phytochemicals found in herbal extracts can be absorbed through the mucosa in your mouth. Putting the extract under your tongue for several seconds will allow some of the herb's beneficial phytochemicals to be directly absorbed into the bloodstream via sublingual osmosis. Some problems—and some solutions—associated with this process will be discussed later in this chapter.

Absorption of most micronutrients isn't usually a problem. The fact that most Americans are malnourished when it comes to several key micronutrients is testament to inadequate diets. However, problems can arise if you improperly supplement your diet. Overloading on one vitamin or mineral can block absorption of another, leading to deficiency in that particular micronutrient.

One particularly relevant example of this micronutrient interplay is seen with the B-complex vitamins (see the glossary for a description). Each of these vitamins can only work if all are present together in a rather precise ratio. In fact, a deficiency in one of the B-complex vitamins results in a deficiency in all the others.

You must steadily regulate supplementation throughout the day so no one nutrient blocks absorption of another. In other words, don't indiscriminately take a handful of supplements all at once, which is known as the shotgun approach. Instead, take the time to read labels and follow directions! Usually, you should take micronutrients—tablets or capsules of vitamins and minerals—20 minutes before each meal so they'll be liberated into the stomach and absorbed with your meal.

Improved Digestion Through Proper Eating

Simply making sure you include the basic food groups and all the proper supplements isn't going to cut it. Eating one, two, or even three large meals daily places your digestive system under extreme duress, and the process is impeded to the point where your nutritional status takes a beating. So, as stated so many times throughout this and the previous chapter, the first and most important step in improving your digestive capabilities is following the five steps of proper nutrition as outlined in Chapter 3.

Besides these important rules, you can take some other steps to enhance the digestive process:

- Eat slowly and chew your food thoroughly. This will allow you to break up large particles, mix your food with saliva to make it softer, and allow the digestive enzymes to work on the starches in your food.
- Eat while calm. Nervousness can affect the movements of the digestive system and cause gastrointestinal disturbances.
- Allow two and a half or three hours for digestion before eating anything else, including snacks. Strenuous physical activity should be avoided for nearly an hour after eating—longer if the meal was large.
- Avoid foods that may irritate the stomach, such as hot, spicy foods and alcohol.
- Maintain an upright posture. Avoid eating while lying down.
- Consult a doctor if you think you have a digestive disorder.

Herbs That Improve Digestive Capabilities

Herbal remedies are helpful in ameliorating inflammations and other reactions that plague most people, including athletes. Soothing demulcents, healing astringents, and general toning of bitters does much to reverse damage. However, the healing process—not to mention improved growth and repair for peak performing athletes—must involve changing dietary indiscretions as well as lifestyle. A number of herbs are of value in helping the digestive system do its job optimally.

A single herb such as ginger or valerian root can change the digestive process for the better. However, combining several herbs can allow each herb to work better. Here is an herbal bitters extract formula designed to enhance the entire digestive and absorption process: ginger, gentian root, bitter orange, dandelion, angelica, rhubarb, cardamon, valerian root, and licorice. Take 2–4 ml of this extract fifteen minutes before each meal (5 ml equals approximately 1 teaspoonful of liquid).

Ginger (*Zingiber officinale*) is native to India, Israel, China, and Nigeria. The aromatic essential oils, antioxidants, and the pungent oleoresins found in ginger have historically had several uses. Recent research has confirmed that ginger is more effective at treating motion sickness and nausea than many prescribed drugs. In fact, a study was done where subjects were given either ginger, dimenhydinate (motion-sickness and antinausea drug), or a placebo, and were then spun around in a chair. Ginger proved to be more effective than dimenhydinate in reducing motion-sickness symptoms in this test! Other benefits of ginger include improving capillary permeability, reducing the cholesterol absorption in the gut, reducing inflammation, reducing nausea from stomach upset, and improving cardiovascular functioning.

Gentian root (*Gentiana lutea*) is one of the strongest bitters known. This herb, native to southern and central Europe, is the standard against which all other herbal bitters is measured. It has been shown to be an excellent treatment against several forms of digestive diseases, including dyspepsia. Gentian root has also been clinically shown to stimulate the digestive system to secrete digestive juices for faster and more complete food digestion, absorption, and assimilation. When taken a half hour before meals, gentian can increase digestive-juice activity in the stomach and provide for better digestion of fats and proteins. (Many experts believe that people with high blood pressure and also expectant mothers should avoid this herb.)

Bitter orange (actually orange peel) contains carminative oils, which stimulate intestinal peristalsis, the wavelike contractions that promote food passage through the intestinal tract as well as the expulsion of gas that causes indigestion.

The next time you pull those familiar dandelion weeds out of your lawn, don't just chuck them unceremoniously into the trash. Eat them instead! Among the most common herbs, dandelions are unequaled in promoting the liver's production of bile, the fluid secreted into the small intestine to break down dietary fat. Studies have shown that use of this herb can increase bile secretion more than 50 percent. Clinical observations have shown that people with colitis, liver congestion, gallstones, and other liver dysfunction can benefit from this herb. Dandelion also contains insulin, a form of carbohydrate, which can help regulate sugar metabolism, making insulin useful for diabetics. Dandelions are also effective as diuretics, mild laxatives, and for treatment of fungus infections. They enhance adrenal function and help prevent anemia by strengthening the blood. The greens, flowers, and root juices are all beneficial, but the root juices have the most medicinal punch. Dandelion greens, more nutritious than spinach, can be eaten raw or steamed and are rich in iron.

Found in a variety of places, angelica has a reputation of being a powerful carminative, soothing an upset stomach, and improving gastrointestinal function. More recently, it has been used to aid those suffering from anorexia. Furthermore, when combined with other herbs, angelica has been shown to have anticancer properties.

Rhubarb is native to China and Tibet as well as other places where it was used primarily for ornamental purposes. It also has been used as a mild stimulant for the lower gastrointestinal tract, as an appetite stimulant, and to aid in preventing anemia. It has been used in combination with other herbs as a mild laxative. Along with its use as a laxative, rhubarb has been used for more than 1,700 years to stop digestive tract bleeding, and it also has antibiotic properties.

Cardamom (*Elettaria cardomomum*) is cultivated in tropical areas. This herb acts as a digestive stimulant as well as a blood thinner.

Valerian root has been used historically as a mild, natural sedative, and for its ability to aid in mental concentration and improved coordination. Its calming effect also seems to aid digestion.

Licorice root is one of the most biologically active herbs known. Volumes of research have supported the use of licorice root in preventing stomach ulcers, in reducing cholesterol levels, as a stimulant for the liver and circulatory system, for anti-inflammatory and anti-arthritic properties, and for the beneficial effect it has on the gastrointestinal tract by inhibiting gastric acid secretion. The list of historical uses for licorice goes on and on.

Other Herbs for Digestion and Assimilation

Cayenne is one of the more popular herbs. It is used as a general stimulant for the gastrointestinal and cardiovascular systems. It's an appetite stimulant; it increases the flow of saliva and other digestive juices, and increases the rate and efficiency of nutrient absorption.

Cayenne can either prevent, cause, or exacerbate ulcers. You should gradually build your tolerance for it over a period of several months. Ingestion of too much too quickly can irritate the stomach and intestines and worsen or create ulcerations. Frequent users, on the other hand, display greater resistance to ulcers and other gastrointestinal problems. Athletes who are almost always on high-protein, low-fat diets have a much higher tolerance for the herb.

Peppermint, and to a lesser extent spearmint and cornmint, are among the most popular herbs; their many uses as flavoring ingredients are well-known. But they are also excellent aids for digestion, gas, and bile flow, and in healing the stomach and liver. The active constituents found in peppermint's essential oil are mainly menthol and carvone. The oil's digestion-enhancing properties have been experimentally verified; experiments conducted in Russia showed improved bile output and gallbladder contraction, both of which stimulate improved digestion.

The aromatic volatile oils found in calmatives reduce inflammation in the intestinal walls. By doing this, they promote proper functioning of the digestive system, relieve intestinal pain, and remove gas. Calmatives' effects on the digestive system will promote better absorption of the nutrients you may need as well as help relieve the upset stomach you have before competition. Fennel and rosemary are a couple of herbs that have calmative effects.

Like calmatives, carminatives have strong effects on the digestive system. They ease gas, indigestion, and intestinal cramping and can also stimulate appetite. Cumin, fennel, ginger, and peppermint are a few carminatives.

Digestive Enzymes

There are six classes of enzymes involved in food digestion that form the digestive substances in your body. While enzymes are not herbs, their secretion and respective actions are believed to be greatly enhanced by several classes of herbal digestive aids. For example:

- Proteases such as renin and pepsin aid in breaking down the bonds between amino acids and proteins.
- Lipase is a fat-splitting enzyme which causes the hydrolysis of fats into glycerin and fatty acids.
- Bromelain, another protease found in abundance in the pineapple plant, is a milk-clotting enzyme.
- Papain is a mixture of enzymes. Its chief function is digesting protein and it is often referred to as "vegetable pepsin" because it contains enzymes similar to pepsin.
- Betaine hydrochloride, a complex of betaine and hydrochloride, is used by humans as a gastric acidifier, which is important in digestion.
- Amylase is an enzyme responsible for aiding in the digestion of starches, glycogen, and other simple carbohydrates into glucose and maltose.
- Cellulase breaks down the tough fibrous cell walls of plant foods, thereby allowing you to digest, absorb, and assimilate the contents of the plant cells more efficiently and completely. An added benefit is that there will be less undigested food entering your colon where it would be subject to attack by putrefactive bacteria.

Bypassing Normal Digestive Processes

The biggest drawback of ingesting herbs and other nutrients we normally classify as nutritional supplements is that not all the ingested nutrient is assimilated. Aside from the wasted money, the level of biological effect you may expect is often reduced considerably. This is because tablets and capsules cannot be tolerated by many people, thereby depriving them of the advantages of herbs and other nutritional supplements. Additionally, it is not uncommon for up to 95 percent of the nutrients in tablets, capsules, or liquids to be destroyed by the stomach acid and enzyme activity either before they are absorbed into the bloodstream or once they reach the liver.

These problems were the battle cry of herbalists and other nutritional supplement manufacturers during the late 1980s when they began providing herbal preparations and other nutrients in sublingual spray containers. Just a few squirts under the tongue, they claimed, would bypass the destructive digestive processes not only of the stomach and small intestine, but also the liver. They were both right and wrong in their assertion.

While the destructive processes were indeed avoided, the substance being administered would cause a rapid spike in the bloodstream, and then get eliminated just as quickly. There was no control such as a slower timed-release mechanism. Additionally, many substances of value to athletes and fitness enthusiasts are comprised of molecules that are physically too large to pass through the mucosal membranes of the mouth.

Liposomes

Liposomes were originally developed in the late 1980s by the pharmaceutical industry and have been used successfully to target cancer-fighting drugs directly to cancer cells. Liposomes are made from highly purified lecithin and are comprised of complex microscopic lipid spheres (see illustration). These tiny lipid membranes gradually break apart, much like peeling off the layers of an onion, and release the nutrients they carry slowly into the bloodstream.

The saying "It's not what you eat, but what you absorb" reflects the essence of this amazing technology. Clinical trials have demonstrated upwards of 200 percent greater bioavailability than you can expect from pills, capsules, or liquids for such nutritional supplements and herbal formulations as DHEA, melatonin, coenzyme Q-10, ginkgo biloba, and echinacea. Further clinical studies on liposome mucosal-spray delivery of other botanicals and supplements are being con-

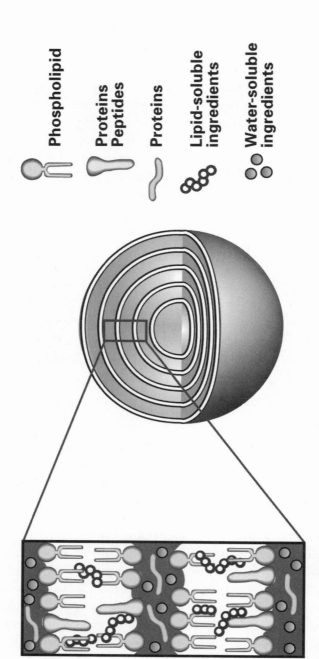

Phospholipid

Proteins
Peptides

Proteins

Lipid-soluble
ingredients

Water-soluble
ingredients

ducted at UCLA under the direction of Samuel Bernal, chief of oncology and hematology, and professor of medicine.*

As a final note, lest you get the idea that this isn't one of Mother Nature's tools, remember that lecithin, also known as phophatidylcholine, is manufactured in your body. It also exists in abundance in such foods as egg yolks, liver, and soybeans. It's rich in linoleic acid, one of the three essential fatty acids. It's principal functions are to supply the body with choline for liver and brain functioning, and to help keep your blood vessels clean of fatty deposits.

---

*For more information on this research and the use of liposome technology with herbal preparations, contact Lifetech Resources, 21642 Marilla Street, Chatsworth, CA 91311. Telephone: 818-885-1199.

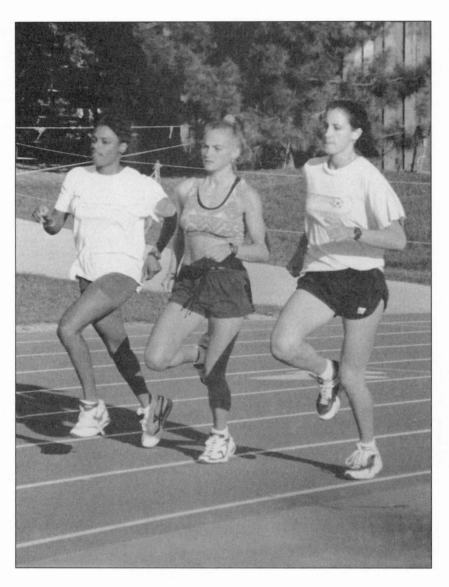

*Even aerobic gurus Drs. Ken Cooper (*The New Aerobics*) and Covert Bailey (*Fit or Fat?*) are now preaching that the fat-loss method of choice is to vigorously use your muscles! It is not merely aerobic exercise! Bigger muscles burn more calories than little ones—24 hours a day!*

5

Fat Loss

"All things in excess bring trouble to men."
—Unknown Roman philosopher

If you decide to enter a race of any distance, would you be willing to carry a twenty-pound weight with you during that race? We're sure your opponents would love for you to do so, but you would be foolish to even try it! Now, apply this concept in your everyday chores and leisure activities. Would you lug that weight around the office with you? Chances are by the end of the day you'd find yourself much more fatigued than you usually are. Then you'll have no trouble understanding why excess body fat is the mortal enemy of all athletes. Even the behemoth linemen in football would rather have more muscle and less fat.

Unfortunately, developing muscle rather than fat is easier said than done, even for serious athletes. And, if we can trust the results of several recent surveys, it has proved nigh unto impossible for everyone else. People in the United States are getting fatter and fatter with each passing generation.

It is utterly strange that otherwise intelligent folks can't seem to break their cycle of overeating and inactivity—habits that are clearly bad for them. After all, isn't it a simple matter of not eating so much and getting to the gym? No, it's not. Research has shown over and over that it is virtually impossible to lose fat and gain muscle at the same time. Therein lies the great paradox. Scientists just don't know how to cope with this problem! Nonetheless, we believe it's simple. If you have practiced a peak sports performance lifestyle long enough, you begin to develop a sixth sense of how to go about it.

The Paradox of Gaining Muscle While Losing Fat

The issue of gaining muscle and losing fat at the same time has kept scientists stumped for years. Here's why:

- While you are consuming fewer calories than are required for body-weight maintenance, you will lose fat. Because you are slowly starving, you will also lose muscle tissue.
- While consuming more calories than are required for body-weight maintenance, you will gain fat. Because you are slowly approaching obesity, your activity level is going down, so gaining muscle tissue becomes increasingly difficult.
- Exercising while gaining or losing body weight makes the muscle loss issue less problematic, but it does not eliminate the problem.

To prevent fat from getting stored, it helps to have a high metabolic rate. That's the rate at which your body burns calories. Two things will amplify your metabolism: exercise and bigger muscles. The paradox is that you can't put on muscle unless you're in positive-calorie balance, and you can't take off fat unless you're in negative-calorie balance. And, since you cannot be both in negative- and positive-calorie balance at the same time, it would appear to be quite impossible to get bigger muscles while becoming leaner. Fortunately, it's a problem that is easily overcome simply by alternating periods of negative-calorie intake with periods of positive-calorie intake. This zigzag process was discussed in depth in Chapter 3.

But, before we introduce some herbal approaches to fat loss that work remarkably well in conjunction with zigzag dieting, let's further explore the issue of exercising while dieting. Weight training while on a calorie-restricted diet can reduce muscle loss, and perhaps among severely untrained couch potatoes, initially add a couple of pounds of muscle. But this muscle is invariably lost during the ensuing weeks of strict negative-calorie dieting.

Aerobic training presents yet another seeming paradox. While it's certainly good for shedding fat, it also wastes lean muscle tissue. It's as if Mother Nature is saying, "Hey! It's too hard to get oxygen and energy to all of these hypertrophied muscle cells. They are not necessary for this organism's survival. Let's just use a few of them to produce more energy, shall we?" Folks, that's the same muscle tissue that burns calories! Getting more muscle tissue keeps your metabolism high and prevents fat from accumulating! You are actually predisposing yourself to getting fatter by engaging in endless hours of aerobic training. It causes a decided reduction in your metabolic rate.

To illustrate, picture bodybuilders in the final stages of contest preparation. They look in the mirror two weeks before the competition, and when they don't see all the muscle striations they think they should have, they freak. They amplify their aerobic work beyond reason and reduce their fat and carbohydrate intake to very unhealthy levels. They spend the remainder of the pre-competition period in a state of ketosis. They lose fifteen pounds of muscle in the last two weeks in order to lose one or two lousy pounds of fat. This happens to many bodybuilders, despite their use of drugs such as anabolic steroids!

The only way bodybuilders can maintain muscle mass and lose fat at the same time is to follow the five rules of nutrition outlined at the beginning of Chapter 3. Bodybuilders bent on maintaining muscle mass while looking totally "ripped" on the day of competition must zigzag their calories. There is no other way.

Natural Treatments for Obesity

Hydroxycitric Acid (HCA)

HCA—referred to in the research literature as hydroxycitric acid— is a natural fruit acid found in abundance in the brindall berry, the fruit of the garcinia cambogia plant found primarily in India. HCA is cited in research as able to inhibit fat synthesis. Possible mechanisms for this effect may be an appetite-suppressant response due to enhanced gluconeogenesis, which makes one feel full; and inhibition of certain enzymes necessary for biosynthesizing fat.

Gluconeogenesis occurs in the liver when glycogen stores (sugar stored in muscles) are low. The process involves synthesizing glucose for emergency energy from protein and the glycerol portion of fat molecules. The protein for gluconeogenesis comes from muscle tissue, while the glycerol comes from stored fat tissue. This is one important reason anaerobic athletes are warned to stay away from undue aerobic exercise—it's muscle-wasting.

Dr. Dallas Clouatre and Michael Rosenbaum, in their book *The Diet and Health Benefits of HCA* (New York: Keats Publishers, 1990), offer these pointers on the use of HCA:

- HCA is not a central nervous system stimulant and won't result in tolerance or cause the side effects associated with these compounds.
- HCA is exceptionally safe because it influences appetite and energy levels indirectly by increasing glycogen production of fatty acids.
- HCA's ability to suppress appetite is the result of a natural process—the filling of the body's glycogen stores. It is natural in that full stores of glycogen increase the safety signal to the brain that the body is full. Glycogen, of course, is the stored form of glucose, one of the body's primary sources of energy.
- Because HCA works with the body's own natural use of calories, dieters will find a greater degree of variation in effective dosage levels of HCA than is true of stimulants such as ma huang, a natural source of ephedra.
- The minimum recommended dosage of HCA is 250 milligrams plus 100 micrograms niacin-bound chromium taken three times a day 30 to 60 minutes before each meal. This dosage can be achieved by taking 500 milligrams of garcinia cambogia, and is the amount used successfully in three clinical trials.
- Subjects taking this minimum dosage of HCA in combination with niacin-bound chromium lost significantly more weight and reported fewer cravings for sweets, reduced appetite, and

greater energy than subjects adhering to the diet and exercise guidelines alone.

- Hca—1,500 milligrams daily—in combination with niacin-bound chromium gives good results for roughly 80 percent of those using the product.
- Those who do not see results at this 1,500-milligram level should double their intake over the course of a week's time. If they do not see results after a further two weeks at 3,000 milligrams per day, it may be that hca will not effectively work in their cases except at extremely high dosages.
- Likewise, dieters with special medical or genetic conditions should not expect to see the same results as those without such conditions. In all such cases, a physician should be consulted.

Athletes who experience difficulty controlling their weight often have an impaired ability to store glycogen, particularly athletes who regularly train to total exhaustion. Inadequate glycogen storage, in turn, is usually related to insulin resistance. Insulin resistance has two primary causes: (1) the excessive intake of simple and refined carbohydrates, and (2) a lack of nutrients, especially the trace mineral chromium. That is why hca is most effective when used in combination with niacin-bound chromium (chromium polynicotinate). This combination increases glycogen production and storage and inhibits the synthesis of new fat from carbohydrates, hence freeing the mitochondria—the furnaces of the cells where energy is produced—to selectively burn stored fat for energy instead of stored glycogen.

Gymnema Sylvestre

Gymnema is an Indian Ayurvedic medicine that has come into modern use after two thousand years of folklore use in India for diabetes and snakebites; as a diuretic, stomachic, and urinary antiseptic; and for other assorted uses. Gymnema has the peculiar property of neutralizing the sweet flavor of sugar if placed on the tongue prior to sugar. In fact, the common name *gurmar* means sugar destroyer. Most studies confirm the antidiabetic property of gymnema. The plant prevents the absorption and activity of glucose molecules. The word *control* best describes the action of gymnema on diabetes. It is not a cure and does not substitute for proper dietary habits, but its use will significantly help keep blood sugar levels within acceptable limits. It is available as a standardized extract in most health food stores. The normal dosage is 2–4 grams (or 2–4 ml) daily. It is best to take 0.5 to 1 ml before meals.

Spirulina

Spirulina is an edible, bluish-green algae that occurs in twisted and coiled filaments. Its nutrient density is legendary. That is, it has a high level of vital nutrients per calorie. It has been used as a food by the ancient Aztecs and in parts of North Africa. Spirulina is grown in tanks on a factory scale and has the special production advantage that it does not need a nitrogen source as it gets the nitrogen directly from air. It is economic to grow because it derives its energy from sunshine, needing only exogenous mineral salts and carbon dioxide. Available at most health food stores, spirulina is an excellent source of protein and vitamin B-12, making it a recommended food for individuals on a vegetarian diet.

Evening Primrose Oil (EPO)

In at least one study, human patients taking evening primrose oil were found to lose weight, but only if they were at least 10 percent over their ideal body weight. Patients within the 10 percent limits exhibited no weight loss. Conversely, another trial failed to find an antiobesity effect of evening primrose oil in subjects who were at least 20 percent above their ideal weight.

EPO contains high amounts of gamma-linoleic acid (GLA), an essential fatty acid known to prevent hardening of the arteries, heart disease, and high blood pressure. It has effects on cholesterol and on the liver. GLA also helps reduce inflammation and improve pancreatic function. The real value of evening primrose lies in the GLA content of its oil. GLA is an important intermediary in the metabolic conversion of linoleic acid to prostaglandin E1.

EPO is available at all health food stores. It is supplied in gelcaps of 500 mg each, and up to 8 gelcaps per day is recommended.

Acidophilus

Lactobacillus acidophilus are the "friendly" bacteria, also called intestinal flora, that our body needs to have an ideal digestive process. However, all too frequently your colon may lack these indispensable bacteria because of your intake of antibiotics, corticosteroids, rich sugar diet, yeast, and stress. The end result is often growth of yeast (*Candida albicans*). Acidophilus needs to be taken around thirty to forty-five minutes before meals.

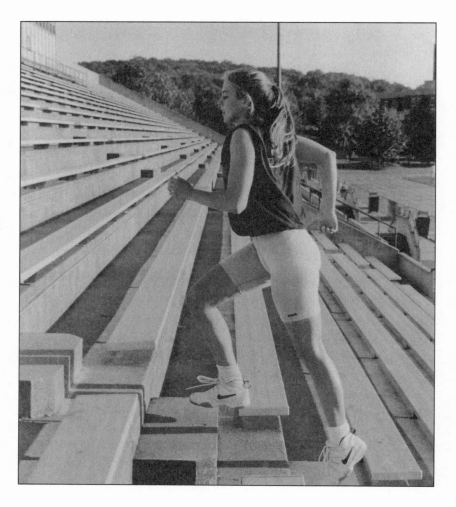

Energy comes from food, right? So, why don't you have enough energy to make it through a game or training session when you're obviously eating enough food? No, energy doesn't come from food—stored energy does. Your ability to retrieve it efficiently comes from grueling, gut-busting training!

6

Improving Energy Levels for Training and Competition

"Fatigue makes cowards of us all."

—*Vince Lombardi*

Physical activity forces your body to undergo both short- and long-term metabolic, physiological, and structural changes (see Chapter 5 on nutrition). There is an inevitable and directly corresponding increase in your nutritional needs (1) to sustain energy for training or competition, (2) for adaptation, growth, and repair, and (3) to maintain normal bodily functions. Let's restrict our discussion in this chapter to your energy needs.

Energy—measured in kilocalories—comes from food. The relationship between food intake and energy expenditure and storage is known as energy balance. When more energy is consumed than is expended (positive-energy balance), the excess is stored as fat. When less is consumed (negative-energy balance), your body's need for an energy source forces it to cannibalize lean tissue or mobilize previously stored fat, typically in that order of preference.

Each of you has a minimum daily caloric requirement we call your basal metabolic rate (BMR). Your BMR is the energy needed to maintain bodily functions such as body temperature, cardiac function, cellular functions, and respiration while you're resting (but not sleeping) over a twenty-four-hour period. (Refer to Chapter 5 for a thorough discussion on BMR and methods of determining your actual energy requirements—your BMR plus whatever energy is needed to carry out your daily activities.) Your BMR as well as your actual metabolic rate are dependent upon your lean body weight and physical activity.

Energy Metabolism and Utilization

The biochemical energy source needed to support muscle contraction is called adenosine triphosphate (ATP). The conversion of this chemical energy source to mechanical work utilizes the energy released from the breakdown of your ATP molecules into adenosine diphosphate (ADP) and inorganic phosphate (P). The problem is, however, that you have limited ATP in your muscles, only enough for one to two seconds of maximum muscle contraction. So, a continuous supply of ATP is needed for longer duration exercise.

To resynthesize the stores of ATP in your working muscles, there are two metabolic pathways, sequences of enzymatic reactions involved in the transformation of one substance into another, which convert nutrients into ATP: (1) the anaerobic pathway, i.e., the breakdown of creatine phosphate (CP) and glycogen; and (2) the aerobic pathway, i.e., oxidation.

Anaerobic Metabolism

When your CP stores are depleted and ATP resynthesis is insufficient to support maximum muscle contraction, glycolysis is activated. This metabolic pathway converts sugar stored in your muscles into energy. The glycolytic pathway is inefficient. Only 22.8 kcal of energy is produced from 180 grams of glucose. This amount of energy is only sufficient for exercises lasting up to a minute, such as sprints, a down in football, or a set in weight training. As glycogen is further degraded, the by-products, lactic acid and phosphoric acid, build up in your blood and interfere with muscle contraction, which results in muscle cramping and acidosis, a decrease in blood pH. That's when oxygen must be introduced in order for muscle contraction—activity—to go on unabated.

Aerobic Metabolism

If there is sufficient oxygen, then aerobic metabolism is preferred over anaerobic glycolysis because of its high efficiency of ATP production. In this process, carbohydrates are completely oxidized to produce almost 300 kcal of energy from 180 grams of glucose. During the incredibly complex process of using oxygen to regenerate more ATP, the oxygen you breathe is reduced inside your working muscles, producing water and carbon dioxide as wastes you breathe out. The process of ATP resynthesis through the use of oxygen is called oxidative phosphorylation, and it's regulated by how much ATP you have in your muscles. Remember, ADP was one of the by-products of the breakdown of ATP.

As ATP is used in your exercising muscle, carbohydrates and fatty acids interact with oxygen (a process called oxidation) to regenerate the ATP. Aerobic metabolism is the primary method of energy production for long-duration exercise, such as endurance events, provided you can get sufficient oxygen to your working muscles.

These energy pathways hold true for athletes and nonathletes alike throughout life. One of your most important training objectives as an athlete is to make these pathways operate at a highly efficient level.

Herbs That Improve Energy Levels

Many herbs which have been used for centuries act as stimulants. In herbology, the word *stimulant* is used to describe an action that quickens and enlivens various physiological activities of the body. This is not necessarily an appropriate thing to do. It's always best to understand what your needs are, what your body is capable of tolerating in the way of stimulation, and especially what level of arousal your sport requires. Too much stimulation in archery, for example, would cause you to miss the target. Sports range in their need for arousal somewhere between blind rage and total calm. Remember that, and you won't have any problems.

In some cases the stimulating effect of an herb comes from alkaloids in the plant. Caffeine is perhaps the best known and most widely used of these alkaloids, and is present in such herbs as coffee, tea, maté, kola, and chocolate. In fact, the coca tree—the source of cocaine—contains alkaloids. Herbalists usually combine such alkaloid-bearing herbs with nervine tonics or relaxants to balance out overactivity.

In regard to improving energy, it should be remembered that no one system of the body works independently from the others. When you improve your digestive, circulatory, and respiratory systems, for example, you inevitably will have more nutrients delivered throughout your body, and therefore, you will have more energy. This chapter lists some herbs which have a direct effect on energy levels, but to truly optimize your energy levels, pays attention to the other chapters as well.

Caffeine

Caffeine is considered a drug, being one of many of the methyl derivatives of xanthine. Because xanthines occur naturally in more than 60 plants, they are found in so many over-the-counter preparations and foods that it's been nearly impossible for the IOC and other sport governing bodies to legislate against their use by athletes. Caffeine, the most potent of the xanthines, is found in coffee, tea, chocolate, many soft drinks, analgesics, and diet aids.

There is no doubt about the efficacy of caffeine in aiding sports performance. Caffeine works. It is known to stimulate the central nervous system, mobilize various hormones and tissue substrates that are involved in metabolic processes, improve muscle contraction, and improve the mobilization and utilization rates of fats and carbohydrates for energy.

Depending upon how strong you brew your coffee, you can expect each eight-ounce cup to contain from 60 milligrams (weak coffee) to as much as 80 milligrams of caffeine (strong coffee). So if you drink four cups of strong coffee daily, and you weigh 175 pounds (approximately 80 kilograms), you'll ingest approximately 320 milligrams of caffeine, or 4 grams per kilogram of body weight.

But—and this is a big but—how you use it is of critical importance in whether it'll yield maximum performance benefits for you.

- Explosive-power athletes—those who do short-duration sports such as lifting, sprints, etc.—appear not to benefit from caffeine use.
- Endurance athletes—long-distance cyclists, runners, swimmers, etc.—can improve their performance with caffeine use.
- Reaction time can be improved with caffeine use.
- Heavy coffee drinkers (two to six cups per day) experience increased reaction time when they resume using caffeine after forced abstinence.
- Administering caffeine to heavy users decreases their reaction time and relieves anxiety.
- The best dose of caffeine is about 3 milligrams per kilogram of body weight. Below that, little performance improvement is noted, and above that, there will be a performance decrement.
- Administering caffeine to an athlete who has abstained from it for several days results in improved performance.
- Improved uptake of free fatty acids by the muscle cells and enhanced use of muscle triglycerides are responsible for improved performance in endurance sports. The net effect of the above functions is that an overall glycogen-sparing process occurs.
- Fat loss with exercise is increased when caffeine is taken prior to exercise (2.5 to 3 milligrams per kilogram body weight).
- The half-life of caffeine in your blood is about two to two and a half hours. Its ergogenic effects, therefore, are of similar duration.
- Because caffeine penetrates the blood-brain barrier, it exerts a powerful influence upon the sensorimotor cortex of the brain. This results in increased alertness, reduced drowsiness, and a reduced perception of fatigue.

With these above considerations in mind, it would seem beneficial to use caffeine before training or competition in most sports, even those requiring power, strength, or skill. Endurance capabilities seem most responsive to caffeine use, but other athletes may benefit from improved alertness and reaction time. This may be especially true for athletes such as power lifters, weightlifters, wrestlers, and decathletes who engage in multiple competitions over an extended period of time.

Again, however, not everyone responds well to caffeine ingestion. Costill et al. (1978) noted that about 20 percent of the population will exhibit enough adverse effects from caffeine as to preclude its use as an ergogenic aid. DeVries (1974) found that caffeine can negatively affect carbohydrate and protein metabolism. Other adverse effects of caffeine include cardiac arrhythmia, excessive urination, insomnia, withdrawal headaches, and "caffeineism," anxiety indistinguishable from neurosis. People with ulcers are cautioned against using caffeine because it causes a 400 percent increase in acid levels in the gut. If you're in the 20 percent who cannot tolerate caffeine, forget about it! The small kick you get from it isn't worth the side effects.

Recommended dose of caffeine as a ergogenic aid is about two cups of black coffee ingested one hour before the athletic event. Don't use caffeine with niacin because niacin has the opposite effect on fat metabolism. Niacin blocks fatty acid release from fat cells; niacinamide doesn't have this effect.

Remember, the most effective dosage varies considerably from athlete to athlete.

Yerba Maté

An extract from the South American plant yerba maté is used widely throughout world to increase mental clarity. Yerba maté (*Ilex paraquenis*) contains a huge amount of mateina, which is related to caffeine but produces none of the latter's undesirable side effects. In addition to being packed also with sizable portions of vitamins B-1, B-2, and C, yerba maté has antistress properties and aids nervous tissue function.

In the Guarani Indian herbal medicine, this herb is used for a variety of reasons, including as an immune-system booster, blood cleanser, nervous system stimulant, hair tonic, antifatigue agent, and stress reducer.

Surgeons in Spain and some South American countries use yerba maté before performing operations. It is recommended as a drink or in capsule form before workouts or competition. Yerba maté has no medical contraindications, even with lifelong consumption.

As previously explained, caffeine has been shown to benefit performance and endurance in activities lasting 90 minutes or more. This effect is related to caffeine's ability to stimulate the release of fats in the blood, which the muscles can use for energy in place of glycogen, thereby sparing glycogen for later use. Exercise experts tend not to recommend caffeine, however, because overconsumption can lead to nervousness, sleeplessness, anxiety, dehydration, and irregular heartbeat.

Yerba maté contains a stereo-isomer of caffeine's molecular structure and provides the same benefits with few of the negative side effects. It is recommended that yerba maté be used three times a day. Water is poured over 2 to 4 grams of dried leaves for a hot or cold tea.

Ma Huang (China) or Somalata (India)

Known scientifically as *Ephedra sinica* or *Ephedra equisetina*, ma huang, or somalata, is one of the strongest herbal stimulants, with an action like adrenaline. Found in Eastern Asia, ma huang has been shown to be useful as a vasodilator, hypertensive, circulatory stimulant, and as an anti-allergic.

Ma huang is a powerful bronchodilator and is the source of ephedrine, one of the main medicines used to treat asthma attacks. It is extremely useful for its nasal decongestant properties as well. Ephedrine is found in numerous over-the-counter decongestants. Ma huang has additional properties for reducing joint pain and promoting peripheral circulation. Chinese ma huang has considerably more stimulating effect than the American-grown variety.

Many athletes use this herb in the form of a precompetition tea mixture. It increases heart rate, thus improving the oxygenation of the working muscles. Bear in mind that ma huang and related herbs have been banned by almost all sports-governing bodies worldwide.

Controversy has brewed over ephedrine, the main constituent found in ma huang. Ephedrine has been banned in several states because, if abused, it is very toxic and can produce long-lasting hypertension, nausea, vomiting, convulsions, respiratory failure, and in a few cases of severe overdose, death. It should not be used if you are hypertensive. Otherwise, use 1 to 4 grams of dried stems, 1 to 3 milligrams of fluid extract, or 6 to 8 milligrams of tincture three times per day.

Astragalus

An herb of the pea family, astragalus is a favorite tonic and diuretic of the Chinese. Astragalus (*Astragalus membranaceus*) is said to enhance the body's main energy flow of breathing, digestion, and elimination.

Originating in China, Taiwan, and Korea, astragalus is regarded as particularly useful for athletes who may suffer from shortness of breath. It increases endurance and helps protect adrenal function. It also promotes the efficiency of the immune system.

The active ingredients in astragalus are an isoflavone and numerous polysaccharides which have been shown to enhance the immune system. The recommended dose is 4 grams per day of the dried root (5 or 6 tablets or capsules or 4 ml) of extract.

Ginseng

The root of the ginseng plant, of which there are more than 200 different varieties—some with, others without, medicinal properties—is perhaps the most highly touted herbal substance in the world.

It is well accepted that ginseng stimulates both mental and physical energy. Russian experiments have shown that daily doses of ginseng for 15 to 45 days increase physical endurance and mental work capacity.

The general opinion among modern experts is that ginseng, as the ancients believed, is an extraordinarily versatile medicinal. Research has shown it lowers blood pressure and cholesterol, enhances cell growth and liver metabolism, and promotes the healthy function of the pituitary gland, the body's master gland.

When taken in moderation as a mild tea, ginseng appears to be a safe, mild stimulant for the central nervous system. The effects of ginseng are cumulative, appearing only after regular long-term use as its constituents build up in the body. It is not a pep-you-up pill. Excess amounts should be avoided.

Siberian Ginseng

For more than two decades, Russian athletes have sworn by Siberian ginseng (*Eleutherococcus senticosus*), a cousin of traditional ginseng.

A series of studies by Russian sports scientists have demonstrated the clear benefits of Siberian ginseng to athletes. According to experiments conducted at the Lesgraft Institute of Physical Culture and Sport in Moscow, it increases stamina and endurance, speeds recovery from workouts, and improves reflexes and concentration, particularly in longer endurance events. The only side effect noticed was a mild, temporary elevation in blood pressure among some of the athletes.

Professor Igor Korobkov of the institute, who studied its effects on 1,500 athletes, recommends its routine use as a health tonic to normalize systemic function, and as an antistress factor.

Medically, Siberian ginseng is used in Russia in the treatment of anemia, depression, and cardiovascular conditions.

The active ingredients of Siberian ginseng are glycosides, chemicals bound to sugars. The glycosides are believed to stimulate the secretion of stress-altering chemicals in the adrenal glands that produce a restorative effect.

One by-product of this is an athlete's long-term ability to adapt to higher levels of training intensity. For this reason, Siberian ginseng is referred to as an adaptogen, that is, a substance that enhances the body's ability to tolerate and adapt to stress. Standard dosage for Siberian ginseng is 1.5 to 5 grams per day.

Gotu Kola

Originally an Indian herb, gotu kola (also known in India as brahmi) is regarded as perhaps the most important rejuvenative herb in Ayurvedic medicine.

It is the primary Indian remedy for nervous conditions, insomnia, stress, and disturbed emotions. It is popular for promoting mental calm and clear thinking, and also for fortifying the immune system and adrenal glands. In China it is a frequent prescription for regeneration and is widely used to enhance memory, decrease fatigue, nourish the blood, strengthen bones and tendons, and calm nerves.

Gotu kola (*Centella asiatica*) grows wild in Madagascar, with other varieties of the plant found in India. The asiaticosides and triterpenes found in gotu kola have been historically used to treat phlebitis, varicose veins, cellulite, and edema. Its action is to stimulate the formation of new blood cells as well as strengthen veins and capillaries. Doses of 50 to 100 milligrams per day are recommended and work best when combined with bilberry, silicin, butcher's broom, zinc, and vitamins C, E, and D.

Hawthorn Berries

Hawthorn berries (*Crataegus oxycantha*), native to England, Europe, and North America, are among one of the most valuable cardiovascular tonics known and have been historically used as a cardiotonic and in the treatment of many cardiovascular ailments. The flavonoids found in hawthorn berries have been shown to dilate blood vessels, which helps alleviate hypertension and high blood pressure. Hawthorn berries also contain procyanidins which act as a sedative and antispasmodic. Recommended dosage is 2–4 grams per day of a combination of dried valerian root and motherwort (3–6 tablets or capsules) in conjunction with 250 milligrams of dried hawthorn berries.

Ciwujia

There is exciting new research about a Chinese herb that has been used for more than 1,700 years to prevent or treat fatigue, increase endurance, and boost the immune system. Several research studies clearly indicate that an extract of the herb radix acanthopanax senticosus (called ciwujia in Chinese) dramatically improves exercise performance and can be beneficially used by people doing both aerobics-endurance activities and weightlifting.

Published reports about the use of ciwujia by Tibetan and Chinese mountain climbers prompted modern research into this root.

Extensive research, including studies conducted at the Institute of Nutrition and Food Hygiene at the Academy of Preventive Medicine in Beijing (the Chinese equivalent of the NIH-SS) and the Department of Physiology at the University of North Texas Health Science Center in Fort Worth, demonstrates that an extract of ciwujia produces several significant benefits. These include:

- increasing fat metabolism up to 43 percent during exercise
- changing the way the body fuels workouts by shifting the energy source from carbohydrates to fat
- building endurance and delaying the onset of muscle fatigue by reducing levels of lactic acid, which causes muscle fatigue and irritation, by up to 33 percent
- significantly decreasing heart rate

By facilitating the utilization of fat as a source of fuel during exercise, ciwujia enables individuals to delay the onset of lactic acid–induced fatigue and exhaustion. All the clinical studies were conducted on a ciwujia extract trademarked as Endurox, which is widely available in health food stores nationwide.

Energy Basics

It's clear that a lot of bodily processes—including recovery—depend on your ability to provide adequate energy. Sometimes, however, the reasons for poor energy levels aren't immediately obvious. You must dig. For example:

- Listen to what your body is saying. Chronic fatigue is a message that something is wrong.
- Don't push yourself compulsively. Stop. Analyze your activities and your diet. Chances are there is no single culprit, but rather a host of factors needing fine-tuning.
- Many athletes overtrain in the headlong pursuit of progress. As a result they may suffer injuries, experience slow workout recovery, lose body weight, and develop insomnia, anorexia, anger, staleness, chronic fatigue, and muscle soreness.

- Remember vitamin R—rest. Get enough rest to compensate for the stress of tough physical training. Not getting adequate rest is a major failing of athletes. Rest balances activity, a concept well understood even in ancient times.
- While supplements and herbs can be natural sources of energy enhancement and are considerably safer than chemicals or drugs, the long-term use of stimulants—whether they be natural (such as the herbs listed earlier in this chapter) or chemical—is not advisable.

7

Developing the Ability to Adapt to the Stresses of Intense Training

"Fight for your highest attainable aim, but never put up resistance in vain."

—**Dr. Hans Seyle,** **The Stress of Life**

As an athlete striving for peak performance ability, you must find a way to ensure that your body adapts speedily and completely to the stresses of intense training. It doesn't just "happen."

Stress comes in many forms: physical, mental, social, and emotional. Its impact on your quest for peak performance can be crippling. To train optimally, you must force both your physical and emotional selves to adapt to the stresses imposed upon them, whether they were imposed intentionally or otherwise. Not only must you strive to eliminate the destructive stresses in your life, but you must gain mastery and control over those you cannot eliminate, or purposely impose.

Merely overcoming stress is never enough. All truly talented and well-trained athletes actually learn how to use stress to their advantage. Beware, however! There's a very big difference between adaptive stress and destructive stress. Adaptive stress forces your body or mind to change in such a way that a competitive advantage is gained.

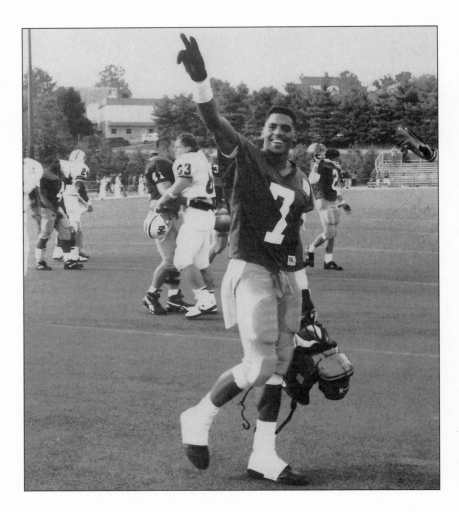

Not only must you strive to eliminate the destructive stresses in your life, but you must gain mastery and control over those you cannot eliminate, and purposely impose.

Destructive stress, on the other hand, causes your body or mind to change in such a way that competitive advantage is lost.

The adaptive process was explained succinctly in *The Stress of Life*, a famous book on the subject written in 1952 by Dr. Hans Seyle. He called it the General Adaptation Syndrome, or GAS. The GAS is comprised of three stages:

1. the alarm stage (application of intense training stress)
2. the resistance stage (when muscles adapt in order to resist stressful weights more efficiently)
3. the exhaustion stage (when after persistently applying stress, we exhaust our reserves and are forced to stop training)

To understand Seyle's theory, think about rubbing your hands on a rough surface. If you do it right, you'll develop calluses. Do it wrong and you'll get blisters. Calluses demonstrate how Mother Nature overcompensates. They are bigger and tougher than your original skin. Mother Nature is helping your body defend itself from your abusive actions. Blisters, of course, are an example of destructive stress.

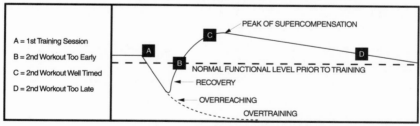

SEYLE'S LAW
A Schematic Representation of the Recovery Process

The General Adaptation Syndrome
"GAS"

Seyle's GAS, when applied to training stress, suggests that an intense training bout causes some bodily systems to function at less than optimal levels for a brief period in response to the stress inflicted. Mother Nature always overcompensates for such stresses by making each system capable of withstanding the level of stress inflicted without having to function at less than optimal levels.

The same sort of adaptation can take place to varying degrees in skeletal muscle, cardiac muscle, connective tissues, and virtually all other systems in your body. It can also take place in your mental approach to the game or training. Mental or emotional stress can, if properly applied, make you tougher and less susceptible to the ill effects it manifests on various body functions.

After overcompensation to stress has taken place, it's time to train at maximum adaptive stress levels again. Generally, this will take anywhere from a few days to a couple of weeks. Continued training at maximum stress levels before overcompensation has occurred can easily lead to overtraining, the phrase used to describe Seyle's exhaustion stage.

By far the most common cause of overtraining is cumulative microtrauma—cellular damage from an overreaching episode that gets worse and worse over time. There are two ways to cope with cumulative microtrauma. You can avoid it, or you can treat it. If you have to treat it, it's too late! You avoid it by not letting microtrauma accumulate! You do this through:

- sensible, scientific training which employs a carefully devised cycle method that allows you to achieve successive training objectives in an orderly, predictable, stepwise fashion
- varying your training methods
- applying the many therapeutic modalities at your disposal (especially whirlpool, heat, ice, massage, and soft-tissue care such as myofascial release or massage techniques)
- practicing sensible nutrition
- using nutritional supplementation and herb therapy
- using good technique in lifting and sports skills
- getting plenty of rest
- taking advantage of various psychological techniques which promote restoration (especially meditation, visualization training, hypnotherapy, or self-hypnosis techniques)
- avoiding all the other stressors in your life that can become problematic to your training efforts (whether environmental, psychological, sociological, biochemical, physiological, or anatomical in nature.)

In fact, you can't adapt optimally to the stresses of your training without following these guidelines. More to the point, you must be able to discern when adaptation has occurred so you can once again inflict adaptive stress on your body, but this time a little more than the last time. This, of course, is called overload, and requires that progressive resistance be applied in your training efforts (see Chapter 3).

Cleansing Your System

Your body is somewhat like your car. You can buy the best quality car on the market, pamper it, make sure it gets the best quality gas and parts, but guess what? You still have to change the filters and oil from time to time. Not because you didn't take care of it. You did. But over time, dirt and grime build up! The same happens in your body. The water you drink, the air you breathe, toxins from pesticides, processing of the food you eat, and the undigested residue of certain foods build up and can hinder your training and athletic performance in several ways.

Your body does a fairly adequate job of removing such toxins. The liver, digestive system, blood, lymphatic system, urinary system, skin, and lungs all work hard to remove as much of the toxins as they can, but for athletes living in a world of pollution and food processing these toxins are overwhelming! The result is slower recovery time.

The first step is to prepare your body for more efficient use of adaptogenic herbs, supplements, and even the food you eat. This is done using a cleansing formula for your kidneys, liver, colon, and blood. The next step is to improve your body's restorative and recovery ability. The final step is to maximize your body's adaptive responses to the ever-increasing stresses of training, the most important parts of which involve growing tissue and boosting immune function.

Cleansing herbs are classified by the methods they use to remove wastes. These classifications include alteratives, bitters, diaphoretics, diuretics, hepatics, laxatives, and rubefacients.

There are many cleansing protocols in use by herbalists, and most of the herbs that are used in them are also available at almost all health food stores. Listed at the end of this chapter is one cleansing protocol that has been used by many of the athletes we have coached over the years. Many athletes feel a bit of gastrointestinal discomfort during the cleansing process, and bowel movements tend to be frequent. Because of this, we recommend that you seek expert advice on this procedure from a sports herbalist before trying it.

Improving Healing, Recovery, and Restoration

You've taken your cleansers, followed the guidelines of performance nutrition and integrated training, and now you feel great! You're in tip-top condition, your body is full of vitality, and you're ready to wage war on the competition! Throughout your competitive season everything falls into place. No mistakes, no losses, no injuries!

If this is your story, congratulations! You are the first athlete EVER who can make such a claim.

As hard as you may try, as carefully as you prepare for competition, sooner or later injuries are going to happen. They happen during competition, they happen in training and practice, they can even happen at home or on the street. Unfair? You're right it is unfair, but it still happens. Futhermore, when it comes to muscle and connective-tissue damage, it happens every time you work out. This is part of the adaptation process: purposefully damage the muscle, then rebuild it stronger and bigger than it was before.

Athletes have long realized this and have sought ways to improve healing capabilities. Your age, sex, and how you eat, sleep, and train are all important to speedy recovery. Each system takes different lengths of time to recover. For example, a good night's rest is usually all it takes for the mental processes to recover. Muscle tissue, depending on the fiber type, size of the muscle, and other factors, can take several days to recover.

What can you use to help your body recover faster? Numerous technologies, training methods, and supplements are at your disposal. You can:

- improve blood circulation to more quickly bring nutrients to and dispose of toxins and wastes around wounded cells
- improve protein turnover for faster tissue remodeling
- reduce the catabolic effects of exercise
- increase or replenish energy stores that help reconstruct damaged tissue
- use sports massage and whirlpool therapy to break up scar tissue and adhesions
- use antioxidants to decrease damage caused by free radicals
- put in plenty of down time—sleep, rest, and relaxation—which your body needs to mentally and physically recover from daily activities and workouts
- supplement your diet with herbs and foods that have wound-healing properties

Antioxidants

While antioxidants are not normally classified as cleansers or adaptogens in the traditional sense, they are responsible for many of the same actions. Normal metabolism, radiation, exercise, ozone exposure, carcinogens, and other environmental toxins cause oxygen molecules inside our bodies to break down. When an oxygen molecule loses one of its electrons, it becomes highly reactive, capable of combining with other molecules in its quest to replace this electron. In this volatile state, the oxygen molecule becomes known as a "free radical."

When the renegade molecule finds an electron mate, it bonds with it, causing the mate to have an extra electron. This new electron makes that molecule highly reactive, and a self-perpetuating vicious cycle begins. Cell membranes are destroyed, immune system integrity is compromised, and DNA—your cells' master regulator—is altered or destroyed.

There are some well-known scavengers of these free radicals collectively known as antioxidants. It has, over the past few years, become scientific dogma that these antioxidants make a difference in your ability to recover more quickly from intense physical stress

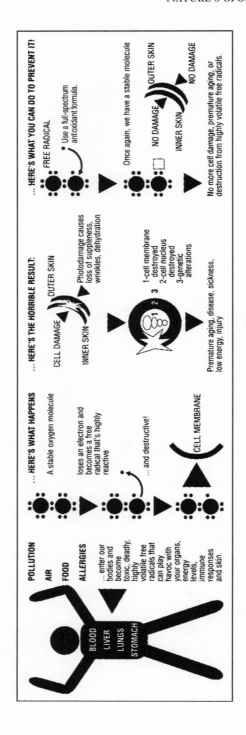

and aid in preventing many of the maladies associated with premature aging.

There is no doubt that free radicals decrease an athlete's ability to recover from training. In the following tables, we have listed the seven known forms of free radicals and some of the substances from Mother Nature's sports pharmacy which may prove to be powerfully therapeutic in your quest for sports excellence. Take them seriously.

FREE RADICALS AND CORRESPONDING ANTIOXIDANTS

Species of Free Radicals	Corresponding Antioxidants
Superoxide anion radical	green tea (GTA) vitamin C glutathione (GSH) maria thistle (assists GSH) ginkgo biloba
Hydrogen peroxide	green tea glutathione maria thistle (assists GSH) ginkgo biloba
Hydroxyl radical	vitamin C ginkgo biloba
Singlet oxygen	vitamin A (beta carotene) vitamin E glutathione maria thistle (assists GSH) selenium (assists vitamin E) ginkgo biloba bilberry (assists vitamin E)
Polyunsaturated fatty-acid radical	vitamin A vitamin E nordihydroguaiaritic acid (NDGA), from chaparral selenium and bilberry (assist vitamin E) maria thistle
Organic–fatty-acid hydroperoxides	glutathione nordihydroguaiaritic acid maria thistle (assists GSH) ginkgo biloba

Species of Free Radicals	Corresponding Antioxidants
Oxidized protein	glutathione
	maria thistle (assists GSH)
	ginkgo biloba

Green Tea

Green tea, also known as GTA (green tea antioxidant) or GTE (green tea extract), has been clinically shown to be as much as 200 times more effective than vitamin E at scavenging hydrogen peroxide and superoxide anion radicals. As such, it is perhaps the most potent antioxidant known to man in its ability to prevent antibacterial and antiviral activity, antiplatelet and hypocholesterolemic activity, lung cancer due to smoking, skin damage and skin cancer due to radiation, and a host of other age-related maladies. The active ingredients of green tea are called polyphenol catechins, with epigallocatechin gallate (EGCG) being by far the most important. Green tea is unprocessed; black tea is the same plant but highly processed; oolong tea, also from the same plant, is partially processed. Stick to green tea. If you don't want to drink it, use an extract or caplet instead.

Bilberry

The active components of bilberries are the anthocyanosides. During World War II, bilberry jam became very popular among Allied forces pilots because it promoted superior visual acuity, especially while flying at night. Both folklore and studies show that bilberry extract protects blood capillaries, protects the heart, shows excellent anti-inflammatory action, inhibits cholesterol-induced atherosclerosis, and inhibits clotting. Its chief action as an antioxidant is its powerful synergy with vitamin E.

Ginkgo Biloba

Native to China and Japan, the ginkgo tree lives more than 1,000 years! The active component of ginkgo leaves are quercetin and the flavoglycosides. Ginkgo extract is shown to reduce clots or thrombi formation in the veins and arteries, increase cellular energy by increasing glucose and ATP, prevent formation of or scavenge free radicals, reduce high blood pressure, promote peripheral blood flow (especially to the brain), and help inner ear problems. Ginkgo also has been shown to improve alertness, short-term memory, and various cognitive disorders.

Maria Thistle

The active compound in maria thistle is silymarin. It is known to improve liver function, help protect the kidneys, promote cellular regeneration via increased protein synthesis, and act as a powerful antioxidant principally through its sparing effects on glutathione (see glossary).

Chaparral

Nordihydroguaiaritic acid (NDGA), the active compound in the chaparral bush, is used as an antioxidant in fats and oils. It occurs in the resin of many plants, particularly the chaparral bush, which grows in the high desert of the U.S. Southwest.

Selenium, Glutathione, and Vitamins A, C, and E

The element selenium is an important constituent of the enzyme glutathione peroxidase. Vitamin E and selenium tend to enhance the effects of one another in that vitamin E works to prevent the formation of free radicals and glutathione destroys those already present. Selenium is an important part of the body's immune system and blood-clotting mechanism. Vitamins A, C, and E are all powerful antioxidants. Natural vitamin E—d-alpha tocopherol succinate, as opposed to the synthetic version, d-l alpha tocopheryl acetate— is particularly effective in reducing exercise-induced lipid-peroxide free radicals. Vitamin A (beta carotene) appears particularly effective in preventing and treating pathologies involving singlet oxygen radicals triggered by intense sunlight. Vitamin C is a real workhorse, both scavenging superoxide and hydroxyl radicals and enhancing the beneficial effects of many other substances in the diet and certain nutritional supplements.

Herbal Formulas

Most health food stores carry several of the following formulas. Look at all of them and choose the one that incorporates at least several of the herbs listed. It is not difficult to mix and match several different products, since they are almost always provided in standardized dosages. Remember that each tablet will usually contain equal parts of each of the herbs it contains.

Herbal Cleansing Formula

Blood and liver cleanse:
red clover
burdock
rhubarb
goldenseal
milk thistle
licorice
dandelion

Kidney cleanse:
cornsilk
couch grass
hydrangea
uva ursi
althea root

Colon cleanse:
psyllium seed
flaxseed

Directions: Take three (3) tablets from each of the three cleansing categories three times daily with meals for the three days prior to commencing your precompetition training cycle.

Herbal Recovery and Restoration Formula

horsetail grass
saw palmetto fruit
fenugreek seed
teasel root
fleece flower root
ginkgo biloba
capsicum fruit

Directions: Take 1–2 ml of the extract three times daily with meals.

Herbal Adaptogenic Formula

Siberian ginseng
Oriental ginseng
echinacea
goldenseal
mumie
pantocrine (reindeer antler)

Directions: Take 1–2 ml of the extract three times daily with meals.

Herbal Antioxidant Formula

green tea extract (GTE)
Siberian ginseng
ginkgo biloba
bilberry
maria thistle
gotu kola
capsicum
kola nut

Directions: Take 1–2 ml of the extract three times daily with meals.

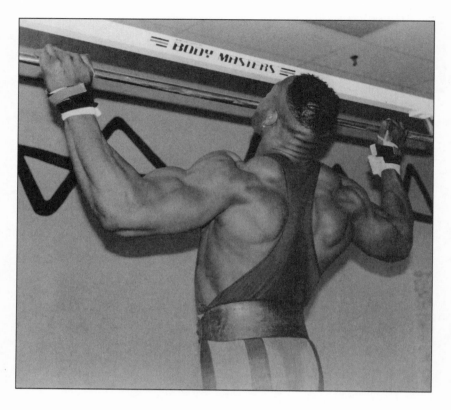

The correlation between muscle size and strength isn't perfect, but it's close! It is also close with muscle size and speed, agility, quickness, and power.

8

Muscle Is the Word for Bigger, Faster, Stronger

Nutritional Strategies for Increasing Muscle Mass and Strength

So much has been written about getting bigger, faster, and stronger. So why don't we see a population of muscular, athletic-looking people out there? Why are most of the "athletes" out there . . . well . . . wannabes?

The simple truth is that while there is a lot of good information to be had, few take the time to apply it. We'd like to make your job of putting on more muscle for greater strength easier. Assuming you're already weight training, there's only one way to get muscles to grow bigger.

Get this straight: nothing is as important to muscle growth as good nutrition! Let's get specific about the most important part of your growth program—your nutritional regimen. When you say you want to get big, what you really mean is that you want to put on more muscle without putting on any fat. So, you have to follow some simple rules of performance nutrition to help you fit your caloric intake to your training and lifestyle needs in a precise manner. (See Chapter 3.)

Maintaining a Positive Caloric Balance

Maintaining a positive caloric intake simply means supplying your body with enough calories for energy, and a little to spare for growth. Everything you do requires energy: eat, sleep, study, work, train, play, breathe, scratch your backside—everything! As you read this paragraph your brain, eyes, and arms (if you are holding this book) are all burning calories. Obviously, some activities require more energy than others.

Your primary source of caloric energy is carbohydrates, which are stored in your muscle cells in the form of glycogen. Once this energy source is used up or is in such short supply that it becomes unavailable, there are only two other energy sources available: stored body fat and muscle protein. Unfortunately, the body will selectively use the protein as an energy source before it'll use stored fat. That means your body actually cannibalizes muscle for energy—and you *lose* muscle mass!

Spread your caloric intake throughout the day, eating at least five meals. This will ensure you get just enough calories to last two to three hours (when you will eat again), and avoid the negative caloric state which wastes muscle tissue. This is not an easy task for some people. Excuses aside, some people simply cannot digest and assimilate food that rapidly.

That's where herbs can really help. Certain herbs from Mother Nature's bountiful medicine chest have been used for centuries for their ability to strengthen or increase the normal function of the stomach. Bitters are an important class of stomach tonics. When combined with other botanicals, they can have a beneficial effect on the rate and extent of digestion and assimilation of food.

Digestive enzymes also have proved quite useful in aiding digestion, absorption, and assimilation of nutrients. Some even bypass the normal digestive processes and head straight for your bloodstream! These and other digestive and assimilative aids were discussed in Chapter 4.

Taking in Enough Protein

Muscle tissue is made up of twenty-five amino acids in different amounts. Your body can produce sixteen of them, known as the nonessential amino acids. You must provide the other eight essential aminos in your diet. If you are a teenager or younger, you need two additional amino acids in your diet, arginine and histidine. The following table lists the essential and nonessential amino acids:

Essential amino acids	Nonessential amino acids
L-isoleucine	L-alanine
L-leucine	L-asparagine
L-lysine	L-aspartic acid
L-methionine	L-citrulline
L-phenylalanine	L-cysteine
L-tryptophan	L-cystine
L-threonine	L-glutamine (conditionally
L-valine	essential particularly during
L-arginine (essential for	intense or prolonged weight
children and athletes	training)
L-histidine (essential for	L-glutamic acid
children and athletes)	Glycine
	L-ornithine
	L-proline
	L-serine
	Taurine
	L-tyrosine

Ingesting glutamic acid with vitamin B-6 before or after training will combine with ammonia (a metabolic byproduct of your muscles' use of protein for energy) in the liver to synthesize L-glutamine. Extra L-glutamine is vital during and after intense training because your body cannot synthesize it fast enough during this period. It's a powerful anticatabolic agent in that it neutralizes the catabolic effects of cortisol.

All forms of intense training cause cortisol to be secreted, particularly running, which involves a huge amount of eccentric muscle contraction that causes muscle tearing. Cortisol is Mother Nature's way of getting rid of damaged muscle cells. You want to repair these cells, not get rid of them!

Many research studies have shown that athletes need more protein than average folks. Approximately one to two grams of protein should be ingested for every kilogram of lean body mass, depending upon your activity level. The following chart will help you compute your protein requirements based on your lean body weight and activity level, or "need factor."

Hatfield Estimate Procedure for Determining Daily Protein Requirements

Formula: lean body weight (in pounds) × need factor = daily protein requirement (in grams)

Need Factors:

.5—sedentary, no sports or training

.6—jogger or light fitness training

.7—sports participation or moderate training three times a week

.8—moderate daily weight training or aerobic training

.9—heavy weight training or aerobic training daily

1.0—very heavy weight training twice daily plus sports training

*LBW (lb.)	Need Factor (protein requirements expressed in grams per day)					
	.5	.6	.7	.8	.9	1.0
90	45	54	63	72	81	90
100	50	60	70	80	90	100
110	55	66	77	88	99	110
120	60	72	84	96	108	120
130	65	78	91	104	117	130
140	70	84	98	112	126	140
150	75	90	105	120	135	150
160	80	96	112	128	144	160
170	85	102	119	136	153	170
180	90	108	126	144	162	180
190	95	114	133	152	171	190
200	100	120	140	160	180	200
210	105	126	147	168	189	210
220	110	132	154	176	198	220
230	115	138	161	184	207	230
240	120	144	168	192	216	240

*LBW: Your fat cells do not require protein, so it doesn't make sense to compute your protein requirements from total body weight. LBW (lean body weight, or fat-free weight) can be estimated using any of several anthropometric, ultrasound, electrical impedance, or underwater weighing techniques.

There are other points to consider when determining your body's protein needs. First, not all protein sources are equal. Some protein sources, like vegetables, don't have all the amino acids you need. You must either get your protein from an animal or dairy source, or eat a wide variety of grains, nuts, fruits, and vegetables to fulfill the amino acid requirements. Second, your body cannot use massive amounts of protein at once. You must maintain a positive nitrogen balance throughout the day.

Maintaining a Positive Nitrogen Balance

The main component of all amino acids is nitrogen. Your nitrogen balance is an estimate of the difference between nitrogen intake and output in the body to measure protein sufficiency. It is derived by subtracting the amount of urea nitrogen excreted (urine, feces, and sweat) from your total protein intake. If you're excreting more than your intake, your nitrogen balance is negative, indicating that you didn't eat enough protein to meet your body's demand, or your catabolic processes are far greater than your anabolism. In this situation, muscle protein is sacrificed to provide additional protein for energy. Simply stated, you must maintain a positive nitrogen balance by consuming enough high-quality protein (high in the essential aminos) to meet your needs.

Beware of how much you take in at one meal. Extra protein is too easily stored as fat. Refer to the previous table to be sure each of your meals has the optimal protein value for you.

Increasing Anabolism and Decreasing Catabolism

It should be apparent that maintaining a positive nitrogen balance at all times is perhaps the most important factor in keeping your body in an anabolic, or muscle-building, state. If you don't, your body is in a catabolic state. This means your muscle is being used for energy because your body could not repair it. Here are some tips on keeping your body in an anabolic state:

• Make sure you get plenty of the branched-chain amino acids. Three of them, L-leucine, L-isoluecine, and L-valine, make up an estimated 35 percent of your muscle tissue. In fact, following intense training, 50 to 70 percent of your amino acid needs must be supplied by these three amino acids. They are also used heavily for energy during intense training. Up to 20 percent of your workout energy can be derived from the breakdown of these three aminos—particularly L-leucine.

• Get plenty of sleep. Growth hormone, which is necessary for muscle repair and growth, is released during sleep. Consider at least eight hours of sleep part of your training. In fact, you can derive an extra growth hormone spike with a 20 to 30 minute nap during the day.

• Avoid eating meals just before sleep or immediately after training. During these two periods growth hormone is being released. Eating meals during these times will raise insulin levels and shut off growth hormone release.

• Consume your post-training meal 45 to 60 minutes after training. This will optimize glycogen storage in your muscle cells, provide your muscles with amino acids when they need them the most for growth and repair, and still allow for growth hormone release.

• L-glutamine, ordinarily a nonessential amino acid, becomes vital during and following intense exercise. It must be ingested before training in order to offset the catabolic response exercise invariably induces.

Training Strategies for Increasing Muscle Mass and Strength

When you think of combined strength and muscle mass, chances are you think of heavyweight power lifters and bodybuilders. By the nature of their chosen sports, these athletes must possess tremendous strength and muscle mass in order to handle the extreme stress of lifting the weights required to achieve elite status.

But the reality is that all athletes require a maximum strength-to-weight ratio in order to achieve elite status in any sport. Basketball, football, boxing—even marathon running—all involve maximum force output while operating within their respective energy pathways. This force-output capability is derived from maximizing muscle mass to a level most efficient for that task.

Look Like Tarzan, Play Like Jane

Many sports require that the participants be as big and muscular as possible. If you train and eat properly for your sport, you can gain as much body weight as you need, ensuring that the added weight is muscle and not fat.

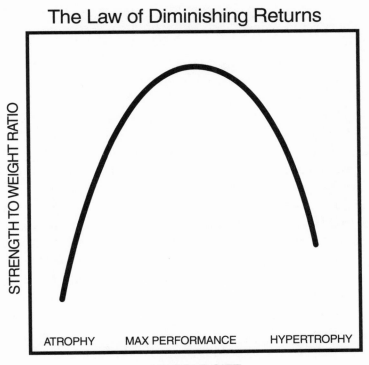

Athletes in sports other than bodybuilding can and often should build massive muscles, but never at the expense of performance capabilities, and only rarely to the same extreme as a bodybuilder. The all-important strength-to-weight ratio must be preserved. That's why you never see a 300-pound heavyweight boxer or gymnast.

All bodybuilders want bigger muscles, of course, and training like a bodybuilder will give you your greatest returns in mass. Athletes in sports other than bodybuilding can and often should build massive muscles, but only rarely to the same extreme as a bodybuilder, and never at the expense of performance capabilities. The all-important strength-to-weight ratio must be preserved. The acid test will always be whether you can perform the skills required in your sport better.

The bigger and stronger your muscles get, the faster, quicker, and more agile you will be. Or, if you're an endurance athlete, the more stamina you will have. However, there is a point for all athletes in every sport where, if you begin getting too big, your efficiency as an athlete begins to go down. You may gain greater absolute strength by getting bigger muscles, but you will lose some of the other important types of strength in the process. For example, factors like quickness (starting strength plus reaction time) and aerobic strength are typically reduced as you grow to a bodybuilder's proportions.

On the other hand, not all athletes need worry about getting too big. Elite aerobic athletes, for example, become elite in their sport by virtue of the fact that they have primarily red muscle fibers throughout their bodies. Red, or slow twitch, fiber has great oxidative capacity owing to the high concentration of myoglobin (the red pigment responsible for maintaining the proper concentration of oxygen in a muscle cell) and mitochondria (the subcellular organelle responsible for the oxidative functions of muscle cells). Red muscle fibers have very little capacity for hypertrophy. The size difference between an untrained and a highly trained red muscle fiber is perhaps 15 percent. The difference in size between an untrained and a highly trained white muscle fiber, on the other hand, can be as much as 100 percent!

Improving Strength-to-Weight Ratio for Aerobic and Anaerobic Sports

The single most important guideline for improving strength-to-weight ratio for all athletes is to cycle your training.

If your sport is anaerobic in nature, and you're in the beginning phase of cycle training, your greatest training emphasis must be geared toward the following factors:

1. a high total number of pounds lifted per workout
2. moderate aerobic endurance
3. limit strength (how much force you can exert in one all-out effort)
4. general fitness
5. improving strength-to-weight ratio, or getting rid of fat and putting on muscle

At the start your lowest output should come in:

6. intensity of effort
7. maximum anaerobic endurance
8. skill and body control
9. speed-strength (starting strength and explosive strength)

But the key to the cycle-training program is to reverse this order of output gradually so that factors 1 through 5 begin to decrease, while factors 6 through 9 begin to increase. At the end of the cycle, you should see a complete turnaround, and your greatest efforts should come from factors 6 through 9, while the least effort is devoted to factors 1 through 5.

However, if you're an endurance athlete just beginning a training cycle, limit strength training, fat loss, and general fitness are still the most important elements of your initial training. Then you get into speed work, hill work, and finally, high-level cardiovascular work.

Anaerobic and aerobic athletes actually train very similarly. The principal difference is that aerobic athletes train while in severe need of oxygen for very long periods of time. They're not working so hard that they can't go on. Anaerobic athletes often train against the anaerobic threshold—meaning that they develop a severe oxygen debt, but they stop when the debt becomes too great to go on. Anaerobic athletes who engage in short, explosive activities (ATP/CP–driven sports such as shot put, power lifting, or high jumping) never encounter such an oxygen debt and therefore have no need to improve their anaerobic or aerobic thresholds.

Herbs to Increase Muscle Size and Strength

If you're looking for that magic bullet so many athletes have come to expect, forget it! Anabolic steroids and other drugs used by some athletes in order to grow bigger and stronger than their God-given ability clearly have great capacity to increase both size and strength, but they're illegal and risky at best.

The question is, are there any herbs or other natural substances or techniques that can give you that elusive edge in sports? Are they worth taking if they're not as powerful as steroids? If you're like every aspiring athlete we've ever met—and we've been down this road ourselves—you'll take every available advantage to reach your maximum potential. It's that simple.

Here's a blend of herbs that can assist in promoting faster strength gains:

> ginkgo biloba
> yerba maté
> blue vervian
> wood betony
> avena sativa (oat)

Directions: Take 1–2 ml of the extract three times daily with meals.

And here's a combination of botanicals which provide your body with both anabolism-enhancing and catabolism-limiting capabilities to make better use of your training efforts and nutritional intake in producing the maximum gains humanly possible in muscle mass.

sarsaparilla root	damiana leaf
wild yam root	avena sativa (oat)
saw palmetto fruit	licorice root
Siberian ginseng	fenugreek seed

Directions: Take 1–2 ml of the extract three times daily with meals.

Also, as mentioned earlier in this chapter, making better use of your food with improved digestion, absorption, and assimilation has advantages in creating a more conducive internal climate for growth. Chapter 4 bears careful study for those who simply can't seem to eat enough to grow without getting fat in the process.

Other Herbs to Aid in Muscle Building and Strength

Alfalfa is one of the most nutritious foods known. Centuries ago, the Arabs named it *al-fal-fa*—"father of all foods"— because they said it made them and their horses swift, strong, and healthy.

As a dried whole herb, this plant is 25 percent protein by weight. It contains eight important enzymes that enhance food assimilation. It is also rich in many other nutrients. Athletes will be interested to know that alfalfa is also an excellent source of vitamin B-6, an essential cofactor in the body's metabolism of muscle-building protein.

Mother Nature obviously knew what she was doing when she created parsley. This member of the carrot family is rich in many vitamins and minerals, particularly vitamin A, of which it packs almost eight-fold the amount in carrots. Vitamin A is particularly important to athletes. It is used by the liver to assemble newly digested amino acids into protein molecules for delivery throughout the body. A vitamin deficiency can result in a diminished ability to build and repair muscle tissue.

Rice bran and other grain brans have been found to contain a sterol substance that has attracted considerable attention in recent years among athletes as a growth-promoting supplement. Gamma oryzanol, as it is called, has been touted as being able to increase lean body mass, decrease fatty tissue, build strength, improve recovery from workouts, and reduce post-workout muscle soreness.

More recently, the basic ingredient of gamma oryzanol—ferulic acid (FRAC)—has been determined to exert an even stronger effect. According to Luke Bucci, Ph.D., an expert on nutritional supplements and exercise, gamma oryzanol and FRAC supplementation programs create comparable benefits to anabolic steroids but with no apparent side effects or toxicity. Moreover, he reports, gains appear to remain rather than disappear once usage is stopped, as occurs with steroids.

The downside is that most scientists—herbalists included—believe there is such a thing as "species specificity" operating here, meaning that plant sterols cannot cause a steroidal effect in humans. Unfortunately, research with both gamma oryzanol and FRAC is quite limited. If further research confirms the promise of initial findings, then no doubt you'll be hearing a lot more about ferulic acid in the future.

Sarsaparilla is found to have a general tonic effect that, like Siberian ginseng, has adaptogenic qualities. The steroidal and glycoside chemicals present in this herb are reputed to act as an aphrodisiac. In some parts of the world, the male sex hormone testosterone is manufactured from sarsaparilla root. Before the advent of Western drug culture, medical doctors used an extract of this root to treat muscle-wasting diseases. Does it work for bodybuilders? Our experience says perhaps, but probably not as a testosterone booster. As with FRAC, species specificity mitigates against such a conclusion.

Increasing Your Body's Testosterone Production

Beyond the question of whether phytosterols can directly increase testosterone production in humans is the question of whether there are other phytochemicals that can do it indirectly. Much evidence exists that this may indeed be possible. In fact, many sports nutrition companies have jumped on this particular bandwagon in a very big and profitable way!

For example, one phytochemical in particular, called chrysin (also known as Flavone-X), is known to be a powerful estrogen-blocking agent. Research has shown chrysin to be nearly as potent as the widely used antiestrogen drug cytadren. Antiestrogen agents in general have the effects of increasing luteinizing hormone LH, which is produced in the pituitary gland and is responsible for regulating testosterone production. As the theory goes, increasing LH indirectly increases testosterone.

There is also evidence that chrysin can block cortisol, your body's natural catabolic agent. Catabolism following extreme exertion such as running long distances or severe weight training is rampant due to the cortisol response. Blocking cortisol dramatically increases anabolic processes which are spurred by the presence of testosterone.

Several herbs contain chrysin, among which are *passiflora coerulea* and balm of Gilead (*populus candicans*). Goathead, however, robs the spotlight in this category. This herb, better known by its Latin name *Tribulus terrestris*, has become widely popular in the bodybuilding community for its ability to increase the body's production of LH directly, as opposed to increasing it indirectly via antiestrogen activity.

Goathead has been used for centuries in various parts of the world to treat infertility and impotence. It was first introduced to the U.S. bodybuilding population as the product *Tribestan*. It is now available in many different products, particularly those including synthetically manufactured forms of the testosterone precursors, dehydroepiandrosterone (DHEA) and androstenedione. These powerful hormones can have some pretty potent side effects, despite their being widely available without a prescription. These substances have been banned by the governing bodies of almost all sports worldwide. A notable exception is professional baseball.

The most important points to remember about testosterone-boosting agents, whether they're natural or synthetic in origin, is:

- There's no such thing as a free lunch! You cannot possibly manipulate hormones in your body without generating cascading effects, some of which can be dangerous!
- If there is indeed some herb-prompted testosterone boosting going on, it's minimal. It won't assist a young man much, if at all. On the other hand, it can greatly assist men over 40 whose testosterone production has waned as a consequence of premature aging.
- Such potions and products are certainly not recommended for women, children, and many others only identifiable by a competent medical or naturopathic physician skilled in internal medicine.

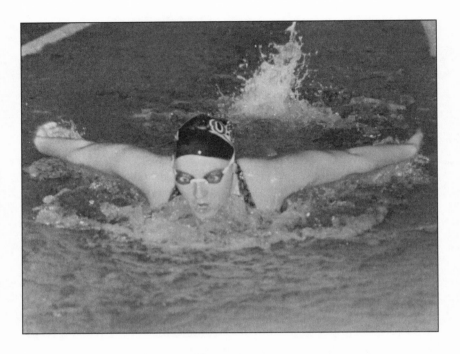

Aerobic endurance—the ability to generate force over and over again while in the aerobic pathway of muscle energetics—goes far beyond mere cardiovascular function. It involves the mind. Are you willing to suffer the intense, prolonged pain caused by lactic acid levels high enough to cripple a nonathlete?

9

Improving Cardiovascular Function

The function of the cardiovascular system has been defined by Guyton (1991) as "to provide and maintain an optimal environment for cellular function." More precisely, it brings nutrients such as vitamins, minerals, proteins, fats, carbohydrates, oxygen, and other important substances to the cells and removes wastes and toxins from the cells. All cells are like tiny power plants; they produce energy for muscular contraction, process materials for growth and development, and dispose of wastes. If materials aren't delivered and wastes removed on a regular basis, cells shut down all activity.

The cardiovascular system includes the following:

- muscle cells—the power plants
- arteries, arterioles, capillaries—the highways, surface streets, and driveways delivering substances to the power plants
- veins, venioles, and capillaries—the highways, surface streets, and driveways removing substances from the power plants for disposal
- heart muscle (left side)—the shipping depot for the fuel
- heart muscle (right side)—the shipping depot to the lungs for disposal

- lungs—pickup site for oxygen and disposal site for CO_2 and H_2O wastes
- red blood cells—carriers that deliver the oxygen to the cells.

All athletes need this important system to work optimally for growth and recovery as well as peak athletic performance. Clearly, athletes in the ATP or CP pathways of muscle energetics need no oxygen to perform their skills. And athletes in the glycolytic pathway of muscle energetics need very little oxygen in order to perform. But all will need it to recover and survive thereafter! So all athletes require optimal functioning from their cardiovascular systems.

Peak Aerobic Efficiency

First, allow us to clear up a misnomer. Most people talk about "cardiovascular efficiency." Indeed, most exercise physiologists refer to the cardiovascular system when speaking about aerobic capacity. They do so, apparently, because it's conventional to do so. Actually, *cardiovascular* includes heart and blood vessels. Nothing more. But there is much more to aerobic capacity than merely the heart and blood vessels.

Heart rate, stroke volume, ejection fraction, and blood pressure all relate to cardiovascular efficiency. Aerobic endurance involves these same factors plus maximum oxygen volume utilized by the working muscles, and the efficiency of gas exchange processes in the air sacs of the lungs. Further, research shows that the greatest marathon runners have two additional attributes which distinguish them from less efficient marathon athletes: (1) willingness to endure pain, especially from lactic-acid accumulation and oxygen debt, and (2) an overall high level of limit strength.

This chapter will explain how to improve aerobic endurance through proper training, diet, and supplementation. Aerobic athletes should carefully study this chapter, but even anaerobic athletes should take note! Anaerobic athletes like shot putters and weight lifters, who often put the cardiovascular system's health low on the list of priorities, need this system to work at peak levels for quicker recovery between reps, sets, and workouts, and better overall health.

Cardiovascular-System Anatomy and Physiology

Heart

The heart is a large ball of muscle which acts as a pump. It circulates your blood throughout the blood vessels and to each cell within the body. It is comprised of four chambers. The right atrium receives blood from the body and pumps it to the right ventricle. From there, blood is pumped into the pulmonary arteries to get rid of a few metabolic wastes and to have red blood cells re-oxygenated in the tiny air sacs in the lungs. Once re-oxygenated, the blood is routed back to the heart and enters the left atrium, where it is fed into the left ventricle which then pumps it into the aorta (the beginning of the circulatory system). It is then distributed throughout the body, with some extra going to the working muscles.

The heart's muscle cells are unlike any others in your body. They are extremely high in mitochondrial mass. Mitochondria are the tiny organelles that manufacture ATP and take care of the oxidative functions of your muscle cells. Because of this, they need an abundance of oxygen in order to continue working. To satisfy this need, the heart is the well capillarized and is the first organ to receive blood.

The heart has a specialized electrical conduction system which allows it to quickly react to stress. Once your nervous system perceives stress, your heart goes into action before you are consciously aware of what is causing the stress. Much like all reflexes found in the body, this electrical conduction system prepares you for action.

Blood Pressure

Your blood pressure is expressed by a systolic reading (the pressure of your blood against the arterial walls during ventricular contraction), and a diastolic reading (the pressure your blood exerts against the arterial walls in between each heartbeat). Along with the heart rate, your blood pressure is a measure of the total work load on your heart. Normal resting blood pressure is usually around 110 to 140 millimeter Hg of systolic pressure and 60 to 90 millimeter Hg of diastolic pressure.

Circulatory System

After exercise has given you a stronger and healthier heart that can do more work with less effort, nutrients and oxygen must be delivered to your working cells and wastes must be removed. Your heart is the pump that makes this happen and your circulatory system the supply line.

The journey of oxygen-rich blood begins when the blood enters the aorta. From there, the blood will pass through your arteries to every muscle and organ in your body. Arteries are lined with a strong muscular wall to assist the heart in maintaining blood pressure. From the arteries, blood is routed into arterioles, a smaller version of the arteries that carry blood to the capillaries serving every cell in your body.

The walls of your capillaries are extremely thin and allow only small molecules to pass through. It is there that nutrients, oxygen, and waste products are exchanged into the cells. Each cell in your body has access to the circulatory system via a capillary. While tendons and ligaments have a very poor blood supply, muscles and other tissues have an abundance of capillaries surrounding them. This makes capillaries the most numerous of all blood vessels.

Both the rate and volume of the exchange of nutrients in and wastes out are important determinants of your aerobic efficiency and your recuperative ability.

Once the nutrients and waste products have been exchanged in your capillaries, your waste-laden blood enters the venues and then the veins. Blood pressure in the veins is very low, so the walls of the veins are very thin and muscular. The expanding and contracting strength of veins is great, which allows the veins to act as a reservoir for extra blood. From the veins, blood is returned to the right atrium of your heart where it is pumped to the lungs for re-oxygenation and waste deposit, to be circulated again throughout your body.

Blood

Your blood carries nutrients to and from all the cells of your body. It is also responsible for fighting off infections and viruses, healing wounds, controlling body temperature, regulating hormones, and overall cleansing of the various organs and tissues of your body.

Though most people do not think of blood as an organ, it is the largest organ in your body.

Tissues

The individual cell is the end of the assembly line. This is where oxygen is turned over to the consumer and the waste products are picked up for disposal. There are all kinds of tissue in your body, including bone, muscle, nerve, and so on, and the smallest unit of tissue is the individual cell. This is the ultimate consumer.

Each cell is like a small factory, with its own receiving and shipping facilities, storeroom, and power plant for creating energy, heat, and new protoplasm—the stuff of which all cells and all living things are made. As complicated as the body is, it's as simple as that. All the food you eat and all the oxygen you breathe is meant to serve this one tiny little factory.

Whether you service cells well or poorly depends to a large extent on whether you send them the proper proportions of food and oxygen on the assembly line. Unhappily, the ratio is usually too much food and not enough oxygen, so the food just stacks up in the storeroom because there is no requirement to burn it. Even if there were, it couldn't be burned without oxygen.

So, when you're thinking of exercise, think that you're trying to pump enough oxygen around your body to fuel all those tiny little power plants and burn all that stored food to keep all those factories in business.

Now, to come back up in size from the microscopic cell, a group of specialized cells together form tissue, such as bone, muscle, and nerve; various tissues combine to form organs, such as the heart, lungs, and stomach; and several organs and assorted parts combine to form systems, such as the pulmonary and cardiovascular systems.

The rate at which oxygen is utilized by all these systems is referred to as "Max VO_2 Uptake." The maximum volume of oxygen your tissues can use is measured in milliliters of oxygen per kilogram of body weight per minute. Cross-country skiers, triathletes, and marathon runners have a Max VO_2 Uptake of 72 to 84. Sedentary people are typically at 25 or so. Other athletes and fitness enthusiasts typically range from 45 to 60.

Training Effects for Your Cardiovascular System

Heart

From your first second as a fetal being to your last breath on earth, your heart has loyally done its job. As with any machine, maintenance and preventive care can improve its longevity. Proper conditioning means you must make your heart work extensively for brief periods of time. Anaerobic and aerobic training raise the heart rate and train it to work more efficiently during rest. Generally, a resting heart rate of a conditioned person is approximately 60 beats per minute. An unconditioned heart may have a resting heart rate well above 80 beats per minute. If a conditioned person was at rest for a full 24 hours, his or her heart would beat approximately 86,400 times in that day. Compare that to an unconditioned person's heart, which would beat more than 115,000 times under the same circumstances! Simply put, exercise strengthens the heart. A strong heart is able to push a larger volume of blood into the circulatory system, thereby reducing the number of times it has to beat.

But that's not all exercise does to help the heart. It also fights obesity, lowers blood pressure, and releases stress, all of which cause a considerable increase in heart rate. With that in mind, proper nutrition and stress management are very important to your cardiovascular health.

A heart may become enlarged by means other than training. It can become enlarged to compensate for weakness caused by inactivity, stress, or obesity. But even though the heart is larger, the individual muscle cells haven't reached their optimal work capacity; their contractile capability is low and therefore cannot pump as much blood as conditioned hearts.

A conditioned heart is relatively large, but its muscle cells are strong. Such a heart is more efficient in pumping blood with each stroke and recovers more quickly. It beats less in all circumstances because each time it does beat, more work is being done than in an unconditioned heart. Even though the conditional heart does beat less, it is capable of beating stronger for longer periods of time than an unconditioned heart. It is much more vascularized as a result of training, which means it gets a lot more oxygen and nutrients than an unconditioned heart. Basically, a conditioned heart has a lower heart rate, a greater stroke volume, and a greater ejection fraction—three factors which make up the cardiac output. A higher cardiac output is what makes an athlete's heart more efficient. Let's take a closer look at the three factors that contribute to greater cardiac output.

Stroke Volume and Ejection Fraction

Stroke volume describes how much blood is being pushed out of the left ventricle and into the aorta, the artery which services all other arteries in the body, with each beat. Although the aortic valve prevents blood flow back into the left ventricle, a certain amount of blood seeps back in. The amount of blood which remains in the aorta is expressed by the ejection fraction and by a percentage. Obviously, the greater the ejection fraction, the better. A conditioned heart will have an ejection fraction of 95 percent, while an unconditioned heart will have an ejection fraction of around 75 percent. Because a conditioned heart can pump more blood into the aorta per beat, it doesn't have to beat as often, which results in a lower heart rate.

Heart Rate

Having a higher stroke volume plays a major role in lowering your heart rate. Distance runners and cross-country skiers, due to their intense aerobic training, boast the lowest resting heart rates. Some have resting heart rates as low as 35 beats per minute! But even a weightlifter will have a lower heart rate than a sedentary person. The fact is, any exercise program will lower your heart rate. The training effect will not only lower your resting heart rate, but your maximum heart rate as well. Because the muscle tissue of your conditioned heart is stronger than that of an unconditioned heart, it can hold a maximum heart rate for longer periods of time. Norwegian cross-country skiers, for example, have been known to hold near maximum heart rates for as much as two and a half hours!

Circulatory System

Training has many benefits for your circulatory system. The fatty foods you eat have lined the walls of your arteries and veins with cholesterol. As a result, the vessels have lost their elasticity, making passage of blood through the vessels an exhausting task. Along with proper diet and supplementation, cholesterol levels can be reduced, thereby restoring normal blood pressure and overall circulatory efficiency.

Local muscular-endurance training can extensively increase the number of capillaries to your working muscle cells. The obvious benefit is that more blood can get to the cells, resulting in greater recovery ability. But this is not the only benefit. By increasing the number of capillaries, you have given your body a larger delivery route and greater blood volume. This in turn lowers blood pressure.

This effect was demonstrated by a researcher who decided to do high repetition training on, of all things, his finger! He constructed a weighted pulley system over the edge of his desk to train his middle finger and began his training program. The first time he found he could do 25 reps, and for several weeks, he showed very little progress. Then one day, literally overnight, he found he was not tired after 25 reps and kept going until he reached 100! Throughout his "finger training" he occasionally invited a mechanic to a contest of middle finger strength. The mechanic, having strong hands, always beat him —until the overnight metamorphosis had occurred. The researcher concluded that rather than one or two new capillaries forming after each training session, a whole network formed, achieving closure all at once!

Blood

The molecules in the blood which are directly related to athletic training are those responsible for transporting oxygen—the hemoglobin or red blood cells. Training has an important effect on these cells. Training increases overall blood volume as well as the number of hemoglobin available. Blood volume in trained individuals has been shown to be approximately a quart greater than the blood volume of unconditioned individuals. More blood and hemoglobin means more oxygen to the cells, which increases their recovery ability. More blood also means a more efficient waste-removal system.

There is another important training effect on the blood, which relates to fat metabolism. Following a meal loaded in fat, that fat circulates in your bloodstream for hours. Eventually it will find its resting place in the fat cells or along the walls of your blood vessels. As noted earlier, this buildup results in the diminishing vaso-elasticity of your vessels and a reduction in the diameter of your vessels, making your heart work harder. It also can clog the area where arterioles and capillaries branch off each other, resulting in less blood getting to your working cells, particularly in your extremities.

The training effect helps reduce fat that remains in your bloodstream by increasing fat metabolism. Effects of fat metabolism were studied in several male volunteers, some highly conditioned, some of average conditioning, and some in poor condition. The men fasted overnight to eliminate interference from other foods, and in the morning each consumed a pint and a half of heavy cream. Every few hours a blood sample was taken to see how fast the fat was being eliminated from the bloodstream. The fat in the well-conditioned males was metabolized within a few hours, while it took the poorly conditioned males 10 hours or more to eliminate the fat from their bloodstreams!

SUMMARY OF TRAINING EFFECTS ON THE CARDIOVASCULAR SYSTEM

Heart	Circulatory System	Blood
Strengthens cardiac muscle tissue.	Reduces cholesterol.	Increases amount of available blood.
Reduces stress.	Lowers blood pressure.	Increases hemoglobin count.
Increases stroke volume and ejection fraction.	Increases capillarization.	Reduces fat levels in blood.
Decreases heart rate.	Increases overall blood supply.	Increases immune competence to ward off infection or other invading organisms.
Increases blood supply to the heart.	Improves recovery ability of all cells.	
Improves overall health and longevity.		
Improves recuperative ability following stress, injury, or illness.		

Herbal Support for Athletes

The following herbs provide an effective cardiac tonic:

hawthorn
garlic
yarrow
borage
motherwort
ginkgo biloba
una de gato
onion

Directions: Take 2–4 ml of the extract two times daily with meals.

Hawthorn

Originating in England, Europe, and North America, the berries of the small thorny hawthorn tree are a most valuable cardiovascular tonic. The berries are rich in flavonoids, which have been clinically shown to dilate the blood vessels of the heart, relieving hypertension and high blood pressure. Since there is no known toxicity, herbalists suggest using 250 milligrams per day.

Garlic and Onions

Garlic and onions have an international reputation as a remedy for lowering blood pressure and generally improving the health of the cardiovascular system. A recent study was conducted on two groups, one consisting of twenty healthy volunteers who were fed garlic for six months, and the other of sixty-two patients with coronary heart disease and raised serum cholesterol. Beneficial changes were found in all involved and reached a peak at the end of eight months. The improvement in cholesterol levels persisted throughout the two months of clinical follow-up. The clinicians concluded that the essential oil of garlic possessed a distinct fat-reducing action in both healthy people and patients with coronary heart disease.

Garlic and onions also possess the ability to reduce the tendency for unnecessary clotting to occur within the blood vessels. They appear to work on the stickiness of blood platelets, reducing aggregation and inhibiting the release of clotting factors in the blood. This is thought to be a property of allicin, a unique thiosulfenate in garlic, well-known for its strong antibiotic and antifungal properties.

Traditional use of garlic and onions in the treatment of hypertension is supported by research. Interestingly, the blood pressure–normalizing and cholesterol-lowering action of garlic is not lost in cooking, while the antimicrobial effects appear to be.

Yarrow

Native to Europe, North America, northern Asia, and southern Australia, yarrow has a high concentration of unsaturated fatty acids which aid the heart by lowering blood cholesterol and may prevent heart disease. Yarrow can be used safely up to three times per day at doses of two to four grams of dried herb, as a tea made from one tablespoon of dried herb, or at doses of two to four milligrams of fluid extract.

Borage

Borage can be found in Europe and northern Africa. Borage has not been used historically because comfrey contains all the active ingredients borage does, and in greater concentrations. Recently, however, comfrey has been found to have a high level of toxicity, whereas borage is relatively safe. Borage contains gamma-linoleic acid (GLA), which helps the body convert linoleic acid into prostaglandin E1. This conversion is easily blocked by several outside sources including viruses, cholesterol, and alcohol. Allowing this conversion to take place decreases blood cholesterol levels and lowers blood pressure. One tablespoon of dried herbs up to three times per day is a safe dosage of borage.

Motherwort

Motherwort is found in central Asia and the United States and grows mainly along roadsides, fences, and pathways. Often compared to valerian root for its hypotensive and sedative properties, recent studies have concluded that motherwort is as much as three times more powerful than valerian root as a hypotensive and cardiac tonic. The active ingredient in motherwort seems to be an alkaloid called leonurin. Because it has sedative and hypotensive properties, it may be wise to avoid motherwort when using drugs which act on the central nervous system. Other than this concern, motherwort may be used safely three times per day with doses of two to four grams of dried herbs, tea made from one tablespoon of dried herbs, or as a fluid extract of two to four milliliters.

Ginkgo Biloba

An herb found worldwide (especially abundant in China and Japan), ginkgo contains flavoglycosides with a variety of uses, including the ability to help prevent peripheral arterial insufficiency and vascular disease. These flavoglycosides (kaempferol, quercetin, isorhamnetin, and proanthocyanidin) inhibit platelets from sticking together and thus increase circulation to all tissues, including the heart. Sixty milligrams of dried herbs can be used safely twice a day.

Una de Gato

Research on the newly discovered herb una de gato has been extensive. The evidence suggests that this herb works well in the treatment of arthritis, rheumatism, female problems, herpes, allergies, viral infections, yeast infections, and other intestinal disorders. The most important element in the herb is the isopteropodine alkaloid, which is a highly effective immunological stimulant. Another component is rynchophylline, which has been shown to be effective in reducing the formation of thrombosis by reducing platelet aggregation, therefore reducing the risk of heart attack and stroke.

10

Mental Concentration

Success in sports performance can be likened to the practice of Zen masters: concentration is so complete, there is no awareness of concentration. Players must be "one" with their sport in order to execute it to their optimal ability.

You have no doubt been in a situation where your attention was so absorbed in one thought that you completely blocked out all others. This kind of focus can be a confidence builder. The more you concentrate on what you're working to achieve, the fewer distractions you have. Once you begin to "see" success, you consider yourself potentially better than the competition. You clearly see your way to victory. You have developed the kind of total concentration that comes to those who have high self-esteem, self-confidence, and motivation, and are consistent in their training programs. You have learned to apply this sort of laser focus to each rep and set of your workout. Just as poor practice habits lead to poor performance, concentration and discipline lead to success.

Since time immemorial, jocks have used everything from A to Z—alcohol to Zen—to steel their minds for the action ahead. Swigging cups of coffee before a game cleared the mind and stirred the blood of Detroit Red Wings hockey star Brad Parks. Swigging whiskey now and then was the great Babe Ruth's style. Of course, he had so much self-confidence and natural talent he could get away with it.

Some athletes sit quietly and meditate. Studies of transcendental meditation (TM) among professional athletes, for instance, show this popular technique improves concentration by making their minds more orderly and settled.

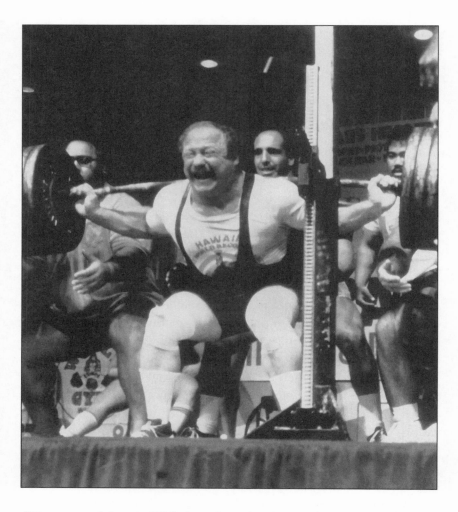

"The power of the mind." Stop and ponder that common expression for a moment. Is it the mind that moves a half-ton of pig iron? Or muscle? Any athlete who has experienced peak performance knows there is another place where mere muscle can never take you. Here author Fred Hatfield hoists a world-record 1,014 pounds "with his mind."

On the wilder side, some athletes have their faces slapped repeatedly or scream in mock anger to create a fierce intensity. Formulas and head trips for mental concentration are as varied as people are different. What works for one person may not necessarily work for you.

Obviously, your ability to concentrate is strongly influenced by the inner "baggage" you carry into training or competition: personality, discipline, attitude, motivation, fear of failure, fear of pain, emotional state, love of what you are doing, goal-setting, anxiety, self-esteem, and creativity in altering training routines to avoid boredom.

Concentration means bringing your thoughts to a central focus and pushing aside extraneous elements so that your mind, in essence, becomes what you are about to do.

To hoist maximum weight, a lifter must exclude conscious thoughts of the movement patterns, the weight on the bar, and the actions of surrounding judges or spotters. Failure to do so undermines the effort. It's called "paralysis by analysis."

Lifters consistently report that record-breaking performances occur without them knowing quite what takes place or having any conscious reaction to their surroundings. The mind seems to have retreated to an inner dimension void of pain, stress, static, and distraction. There is only the pure, awesome potential of all possibilities.

It is easy to see that your ability to focus intensely is a major determinant in achieving peak performance. And it can indeed be controlled! One way that is often overlooked is to control what you eat.

Nourishing Your Brain

Your brain is not some independent instrument operating on a different scale of notes than the rest of your body. Your brain and the nervous system it controls, the muscles the nervous system controls, and the whole ball of wax that is *you* are an interrelated mind-body totality requiring good nutrition to function well.

This totality must constantly be nourished by oxygen, glucose, fats, amino acids, vitamins, and minerals. Muscles are fueled by glucose, the simple sugar broken down from carbohydrates. Yet the brain is the largest consumer of glucose in your body.

In today's polluted and chemical-dependent world, you must eat both offensively and defensively to maintain optimum physical and mental energy. Offensively means emphasizing those foods that will provide you with nutrients to keep your mind clear, focused, and energized. Defensively means learning which foods or chemical additives can boggle your brain . . . and then staying away from them.

Achieving peak performance ability requires that you focus on what you eat if you want better concentration. If you don't, you'll find yourself in the same languid lane of life occupied by vast numbers of Americans whose poor eating habits cause chronic mood swings, mental ups and downs, and lack of concentration. That lane, by the way, includes plenty of unfulfilled and puzzled athletes who can't figure out why they don't get ahead.

Hypoglycemia and Mental Focus

Food is widely overlooked as the cause of mood swings, depression, and the inability to think clearly. For example, hypoglycemia, a condition in which the blood sugar levels drop, sets off a variety of biochemical reactions that affect brain chemistry, causing such symptoms as fatigue, depression, irritability, hostility, headache, confusion, and anxiety. The contemporary Western diet, with large amounts of sugar and other refined carbohydrates such as enriched-flour baked goods, processed grains, and alcohol, contributes to hypoglycemia.

In the treatment of hypoglycemia, many people cut out sugar and refined carbohydrates and experience only partial relief. They may even feel worse—a symptom of sugar withdrawal—or perhaps feel refreshingly "up" for days or parts of days. But the improvement doesn't last.

These people need to do more than just eliminate sugar. They need to add wholesome snacks of protein or complex carbohydrates every few hours to prevent blood sugar dips, or perhaps B-complex vitamin supplements to fortify their nervous systems. The drop in blood sugar levels that creates symptoms is highly individual. A minute dip, deemed normal by standard glucose-tolerance testing, can be troublesome for many people. The persistent mood changes, energy deficits, and lack of focus that develop from low blood sugar over a long period of time generally take about two or three months to be relieved after the start of a corrective program.

Perhaps one of the best ways to control hypoglycemia is by carefully monitoring the rate at which food is broken down and enters the blood as glucose. Nutritionists now assign ratings to different carbs based on how quickly they increase glucose levels in comparison to glucose itself. The system is called the glycemic index.

Simple or refined carbs, including table sugar and many sweets, have long been thought to be absorbed into the bloodstream faster than complex carbs, causing roller-coaster rides of blood sugar. Among the side effects of such ups and downs are headaches, fatigue, and lack of concentration.

As the accompanying chart shows, boiled carrots produce a blood sugar response that is 92 percent that of glucose. Fructose, the primary sugar of fruit, has an index rating of about 20. That means it is very slowly absorbed and converted. Slow absorption is desirable for maximum brain and body function. Therefore, favor foods with a lower glycemic index rating. Fruits and beans are good examples and are also high in fiber.

GLYCEMIC INDEX OF VARIOUS FOODS

Food	Glycemic Index
Grain, Cereal Products	
Bread (white)	69
Buckwheat	51
Millet	71
Pastry	59
Rice (brown)	66
Rice (white)	71
Spaghetti (wholemeal)	42
Spaghetti (white)	50
Sponge cake	46
Sweet corn	59
Breakfast Cereals	
All-Bran	51
Cornflakes	80
Muesli	66
Porridge Oats	49

GLYCEMIC INDEX OF VARIOUS FOODS *(continued)*

Food	Glycemic Index
Shredded Wheat	67
Weetabix	75
Biscuits	
Digestive	59
Oatmeal	54
Rich Tea	55
Ryvita	69
Water	63
Fresh Legumes	
Broad beans	79
Frozen peas	51
Root Vegetables	
Beeroot	64
Carrots	92
Parsnips	97
Potato (instant)	80
Potato (new)	70
Potato (sweet)	48
Swede	48
Yams	51
Dried and Canned Legumes	
Beans (canned, baked)	40
Beans (butter)	36
Beans (haricot)	31
Beans (kidney)	29
Beans (soya)	15
Beans (canned, soya)	14
Peas (blackeye)	3
Peas (chick)	36
Peas (marrowfat)	47
Lentils	29
Fruit	
Apples (golden delicious)	39
Bananas	62
Oranges	40
Orange juice	46
Raisins	64
Sugars	
Fructose	20
Glucose	100

GLYCEMIC INDEX OF VARIOUS FOODS *(continued)*

Food	Glycemic Index
Maltose	105
Sucrose	59
Dairy Products	
Ice cream	36
Milk (skimmed)	32
Milk (whole)	34
Yogurt	36
Miscellaneous	
Fish fingers	38
Honey	87
Mars bar	68
Peanuts	13
Sausages	28
Tomato soup	38

Loss of Mental Concentration Due to Food Sensitivities

Food and beverages are complex biochemical substances, both in their natural state and even more so in their processed state where they are laden with chemical add-ons or contaminants. In either state, foods and food chemicals are troublesome for many people. Furthermore, contemporary mass production strips food of many valuable nutrients that, left intact, would provide protective benefits.

Common allergic reactions can trigger mental changes in the following ways:

- Capillaries leak and ooze fluid, causing tissue to swell around them. The nasal obstruction in hay fever results from such leaks in the nose. In the brain this can cause malfunction among nerve cells.
- In asthma, allergic spasms of the muscles of the bronchial tubes interfere with respiration, causing shortness of breath and wheezing. Similarly, spasms in very small arteries of the brain can reduce the flow of glucose, oxygen, and other nutrients needed by sensitive brain tissue, with resultant changes in concentration, memory, or behavior.

- Loss of stamina, digestive disorders, gas and bloating, headaches, weight gain, visual disturbances, unsteadiness, coordination difficulties, muscular pains, and tenderness in the area
  of old injuries will affect your ability to concentrate.

The most frequently eaten and craved foods are often the most frequent causes of symptoms. Dosage is also important. A particular food eaten once every four or five days may be fine, but taken on a daily basis may develop into a problem. Wheat, milk, corn, soy, cane sugar, and yeast are major offenders. Sensitivities usually embrace all foods containing these products. Thus a person may never eat an ear of corn but may react to corn syrup, corn oil, or corn starch widely used in the food industry. Somebody sensitive to grapes, yeast, and corn can likewise be sensitive to alcoholic beverages.

To complicate matters, some people can cruise along without any signs of food allergy until they experience emotional or physical stress, become chilled or overheated, or inhale heavy environmental pollution.

Endurance athletes should be alert to wheat allergies whenever they embark on a carbohydrate-loading program. Be careful about loading up on spaghetti, a wheat product, or on pizza, which contains wheat and cheese. There are some less offending complex carbohydrates such as brown rice, beans, lentils, sweet potatoes, and even pasta made from artichoke flour.

A general rule of thumb is to eat a varied diet to reduce possibility of food allergies. Try to eat food as wholesome, natural, chemical-free, and unprocessed as possible. To test yourself for a suspected food sensitivity, try the elimination test. Avoid that food for five to seven days. Then take a large portion and watch for reactions over the next few hours.

Amino Acids and Mental Focus

Many of the amino acids found in protein foods are vital to mental concentration. A broad-based amino acid supplement can improve your body's ability to assimilate and use dietary protein, and ensure you have all the aminos necessary for mental sharpness. Among the individual aminos, the following are regarded as particularly important to mental function:

- L-tyrosine is the principal ingredient used by the brain to produce dopamine and norepinephrine, the two brain chemicals related to thinking quicker, reacting more rapidly, and feeling more attentive, motivated, and mentally energetic. In a recent study conducted by the U.S. Army, the effect of L-tyrosine supplementation was tested on soldiers subjected to harsh physical conditions in the field. Compared to a control group that did not receive supplements, the soldiers who received L-tyrosine performed better at mental tasks requiring alertness and were better able to make complex decisions. They also appeared to be in a better mood and less anxious and tense than the other soldiers.
- At the opposite pole from L-tyrosine is L-tryptophan, which stimulates the secretion of serotonin, a brain chemical that has a calming effect. It is used in the treatment of insomnia, stress, and migraines.
- Many athletes use branched chain amino acid (BCAA) supplements to improve muscle mass and endurance. They should always be taken at a different time than L-tryptophan and L-tyrosine because BCAAs can block the uptake of those amino acids.
- L-glutamine is intimately involved with the brain's use of its primary energy fuel, glucose. Glutamine helps memory and concentration.
- L-phenylalanine produces and maintains an elevated and positive mood, alertness, and drive, and also enhances learning and memory. It is used in the treatment of certain types of depression. This amino acid is also very useful for pain reduction in its modified DL-phenylalanine form.
- L-serine is an important factor in the formation of acetylcholine, a paramount brain chemical that aids memory and nervous system function.

The highest quality of the amino acids listed above—also the most expensive—are pure, crystalline aminos. If you can afford the price, buy them. They offer the best biological activity in the body and are more effective for achieving specific results from individual aminos. Peptide-bonded aminos are the less expensive version and are fine as general-purpose multiple aminos.

As an athlete, your responsibility to your brain is quite clear. You require a powerful, precisioned interplay of muscles and nerves, electrochemicals, and enzymes in a synchrony of mind and matter to perform to your max. To muster the strength, skill, and focus you need to succeed depends a great deal on what you put into your mouth. The five rules of performance nutrition outlined in Chapter 3 can help you get more mental mileage from your food.

And do not overeat, especially prior to game time. Research shows there is as much as a 16 percent drop in performance of repetitive tasks immediately following meals. There's also a direct relationship between the quantity of calories you consume at one sitting and subsequent mental alertness. When calories go up, mental performance goes down. There's an adage that says that you should get up from the table when your stomach is half full. It's best to modify pregame eating from preworkout eating by reducing caloric intake by about half. Learn from this wisdom. Stay hungry!

Herbs for Mental Focus

Mother Nature didn't make a mistake by making your brain sensitive to various foods and chemicals, or by causing you to lose your ability to concentrate if you don't avoid them. It's her way of telling you that you're doing something wrong! But she also gave you some rather powerful chemicals to use for improving your brain's ability to function. Many of these phytochemicals can be quite dangerous, causing your brain to work overtime or in rather bizarre ways. Just think about the hallucinogenic and disorienting effects you'd experience if you introduced into your body any one of various forms of mushroom, cocaine, or marijuana. On the other hand, there are numerous herbs that can aid remarkably in *improving* your ability to concentrate.

Caffeine, as we all know, is a stimulant found in coffee, black tea, and cola drinks that can create mental alertness. But it can also create nervousness, anxiety, and sleeplessness.

If coffee isn't your cup of tea, you may want to go the yerba maté route being followed by more and more athletes. Yerba maté is an extract from an Argentine plant used extensively as a stimulating tea drink throughout the Spanish-speaking world. It is highly endowed with vitamins B-1, B-2, and C, and a natural substance called mateina. The bottom line is that yerba maté has a selective effect on the nervous system that enhances concentration. Surgeons in Spain and Latin America use it before operations. You can take it—either as a drink or in capsule form—before workouts or competition. Happily, it does not generate any of the undesirable side effects that occur from imbibing too much caffeine.

Russian athletes have been making good use of Siberian ginseng for years. Studies conducted in the former Soviet Union have shown that it increases endurance, reflexes, stamina, motivation, coordination, and concentration.

Ginseng is regarded as an adaptogenic substance, meaning it helps to systematically normalize bodily functions. It contains active compounds known as glycosides, which are chemicals bound to sugar. These glycosides are capable of stimulating protective, restorative responses to stress. Ginseng has been used around the world for centuries as a natural upper. It is also a traditional herbal tonic for anxiety.

Originally an Indian herb, gotu kola (known in India as brahmi and in China as fo-ti) is regarded as perhaps the most important rejuvenative herb in Ayurvedic medicine. It is the primary Indian remedy for nervous conditions, insomnia, stress, and disturbed emotions. It is popular for promoting mental calm and clear thinking, and also for fortifying the immune system and adrenal glands. In China, fo-ti is a frequent prescription for regeneration and is widely used to enhance memory, decrease fatigue, nourish the blood, strengthen bones and tendons, and calm nerves.

Kava kava is the name applied to an herb South Seas islanders use in a drink taken in their religious ceremonies. The root is chewed or ground up to make a mash; saliva is added on chewing, causing enzymatic degradation to a fully intoxicating substance. The drink causes calmness and relaxation, with enhanced mental activity.

Kava kava appears to be without narcotic action. The active constituents in the root are lactones called kava pyrones: kavaine, dihydrokavaine, methysticin, dihydromethysticin, and yangonin, which, in high doses, depress the central nervous system at the level of the reticular formation of the brain stem, and relax the skeletal muscles.

The Prestart Phenomenon in Sports

Ever get the "prestart phenomenon" jitters before competition? Many athletes suffer to the point that they can't hold down food. No doubt there's a bit of anxiety before competition. Anxiety is a state of uneasiness characterized by worry, apprehension, or fear. It is usually accompanied by physical sensations. Although normal, it can be quite disruptive to your competitive efforts. From an athlete's perspective, here are some typical causes of prestart:

- anticipation of the conflict situation to come
- real or perceived physical threat (getting hurt, etc.)
- real or perceived emotional threat (losing, not playing, etc.)
- stress factors in athletic life
- recent withdrawal from alcohol, tobacco, or other drugs (common among athletes who must play under the threat of being tested for banned substances)

Signs and symptoms of prestart include:

feeling of uneasiness
abdominal pain
restlessness
dry mouth
irritability
trembling
inability to concentrate
fast pulse
insomnia
weakness
anorexia
sweaty palms or face
frightening dreams
nausea
tightness in chest
diarrhea
headache
frequent urination

pain in back or neck
uneven voice

Extreme cases of prestart anxiety manifest symptoms such as:

intense feeling of apprehension or fear
racing or pounding chest
breathlessness
widely dilated pupils
choking sensation
hyperventilation
dizziness
fainting
tremors
spasms of the cardiac or pyloric portions of the stomach

Herbal Combination for Preventing Prestart

One of the best herbs for preventing prestart is kava kava. Taken alone, kava kava works remarkably well at calming jittery nerves. However, here is a tried-and-true tonic that works as well or better for many athletes:

valerian root
passionflower
wood betony
black cohosh root
skullcap
hops
ginger root

Directions: Take 2–4 ml of the extract two times daily with meals.

Aromatherapy

Aromatherapists believe much can be accomplished by setting the mood to train or compete. By inhaling certain smells, they believe you can literally create emotions such as rage, love, calmness, and even disgust. Athletes often smell ammonia capsules before competing. This is common among weightlifters and power lifters who must pull up tremendous aggressive rage before each lift. The ammonia, they say, awakens them and gets them motivated. But there's a better way, and it comes from Mother Nature.

The powerful blend of the following aromatherapy oils is formulated to motivate. It'll do that, make no mistake! When you breathe this stuff, there's an uplifting feeling that somehow taps into your inner strength—sort of like a mind stimulant. When you use this blend during workouts—just before max sets—you'll feel invigorated and motivated.

This energizing and stimulating blend is comprised of a cotton bag containing tiny beads of plastic filled with the essential oils of the following herbs:

lemongrass
grapefruit
lemon
geranium
eucalyptus
lavender
hyssop
bergamot
peppermint
clove
menthol
cypress
juniper berry

We do not expect you to be able to find this particular blend of essential oil, as it was manufactured over a decade ago. Instead, it is meant to be an example of what you may find in the health food stores and aromatherapy specialty shops.

II

Sleep: Nature's Most Powerful Restorative

Sleep is a time for restoring body and mind. It's also a time for growth. Seem obvious? So, why is it that so many athletes sleep less than eight hours each night? Why is it that Americans eschew the worldwide custom of a midday siesta? Athletes must not fall prey to this regressive attitude. There is too much at stake.

To some folks sleep comes easily. To others, not so easily. In either case, once achieved, it induces a veritable cascade of biochemical events that take place all night long in a natural, purposeful rhythm. Any scientifically sound sleep-enhancing program requires at least three important attributes:

- Both body and mind must need sleep before summoning it.
- Once achieved, the multitude of sleep-related activities must be synergistic.
- There must be at least seven to eight hours of uninterrupted sleep.

Patterned deep sleep followed by rapid eye movement (REM) sleep, during which dreaming occurs, describes your eight hours of slumber. Most folks get about four such alternating rhythms during the night. A major spike in growth hormone accompanies the deep sleep cycles.

If you aren't one yourself, you've probably known active people who sleep less than most, yet are wide awake all day, and inactive

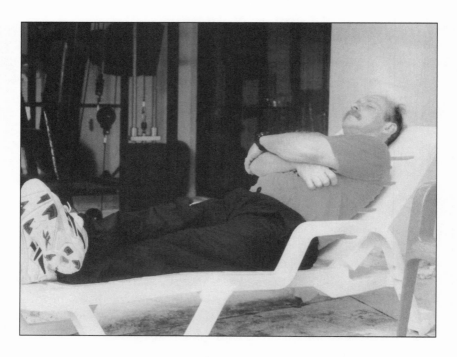

Sleep is a time for restoration of body and mind. It's also a time for growth. Seem obvious? So, why do so many people sleep less than eight hours each night? Why is it that Americans eschew the worldwide custom of a midday siesta? Athletes must not fall prey to these bad habits.

people who can stay in bed 10 hours and still feel listless the next day. This phenomenon was studied using bed-rest programs of differing types with two test groups. Both groups stayed in bed, flat on their backs, for three full weeks. One group exercised three times daily on bicycle ergometers strapped to the beds; the other group did nothing.

The exercise group had normal sleep patterns, sleeping eight hours at night. The inactive group slept erratically or developed chronic insomnia. Some had problems with constipation.

This became a significant study. The Gemini astronauts, especially on the longer flights, slept fitfully. The inactivity involved in weightlessness, added to the normal deterioration that goes on during a weightless state, indicates that some form of exercise may be mandatory for astronauts on long space voyages to help them sleep better and be more alert when awake.

Back on Earth, the same rules apply. If you sleep soundly, you're more wide awake during the day. The listless types are those who usually don't get all the benefits they should from sleep.

Most trained athletes sleep like dead people, and those first getting introduced to a regular exercise program say that sounder sleep is the first physical reaction they experience from their conditioning program. There can't be much doubt that exercise relaxes your body, sleep comes easier, and you get more benefit from sleep in a shorter time.

Just how much sleep one needs depends on the individual, of course. But most people who say "I can do with just five or six hours a night" are fooling themselves. Extensive evidence points to a need for at least eight hours per night, and often as much as nine or more hours. You can get by on less, but it catches up with you eventually. Try it for yourself. Go to bed earlier and get in an extra hour every night for a week. You'll be quite surprised at how your alertness and vitality improve.

The Midday Siesta

"Three in the afternoon. Fading fast. Gotta get psyched! Workout's at five! Coffee. Yeah! That's the ticket! Maybe if I take a walk or something! I'm so tired!"

If scientific research has shown us anything about the ubiquitous mid-afternoon slump in energy, it's that you shouldn't fight it. It's a universal characteristic, it's normal, it's good, and it certainly isn't necessarily due to poor eating habits as is so often claimed. Go with the flow! Take a nap!

In our country, taking a nap—a midday siesta—isn't socially acceptable. Neither is it always feasible if you're working for a living. All over the world people close up shop for a couple of midday hours of snoozola. Not in high-speed USA, though! It's as though taking a nap when your body's natural circadian rhythms beg for one would be considered laziness.

Too bad. If you're an athlete in heavy training—especially training twice a day as most elite bodybuilders must—that nap can be mighty important. Not only will it revitalize you for a more intense noon or evening workout, but it'll provide an important growth hormone response for anabolism to occur, and it'll allow other recuperative processes to take place, making it possible to do more frequent heavy workouts.

Russian sports scientists have spent a lot of time and rubles over the years studying the recovery process in elite athletes. In fact, most of their efforts in sports research have centered on recuperative techniques and substances. Consider the following advice based on their conclusions:

- Take a nap in the afternoon.
- Take a nap in the morning, too, if you can.
- Keep your naps under a half hour's duration. If you sleep longer than that, you'll go into the deeper stages of sleep, causing you to feel groggy thereafter.
- If you work during the day, find a nice shady tree or some secluded spot to grab a wink or two during lunch hour. Take a late lunch if you can—around two in the afternoon would be ideal.
- Never eat a big lunch or drink alcohol during lunch as these practices tend to exacerbate (but do not cause) the midday slump.
- Don't sleep more than eight hours at night. Opt instead for a seven-hour sleeping schedule. You'll find that your mid-morn-

ing and mid-afternoon nap will be sufficient to bring you up to a total of eight hours per 24-hour period.

- If you're trying unsuccessfully to put on some lean body weight during the day, then stay lazy. Avoid unnecessary activity, running around, long walks, or forcing yourself to stay awake when nature calls you to sleep. Remember the lesson from the cattle industry—pen the cattle up so they can't range, and feed them plenty of protein throughout the day—and your muscle growth efforts will be supportively served.

- If you suffer from insomnia (about 10 percent of the population suffers from some form of sleep disorder), taking a nap may not be advisable. Instead, consult a sleep disorder specialist. Chronic daytime drowsiness is most often a function of how well—or how poorly—you sleep at night.

The two most compelling reasons elite athletes don't take naps or practice a more sedentary between-workout routine are (1) they'd be fired, or (2) they'd feel guilty about their apparent laziness because of our social mores. If you can find a way around these two problems—and most athletes can if they really want to—then your training and recovery efforts will surely improve.

Most sleep disorder scientists agree that taking a midday nap can be normal, healthy, and contribute to improved alertness and creativity. Dr. Alan Lankford, director of Atlanta's Sleep Disorder Center, said, ". . . [for] people who, for whatever reason, need to take a nap in the afternoon, there's a payoff in increased alertness and better cognitive function, and they're likely to be more productive at work." That means athletes, too!

So don't be shy! Take a brief 20 to 30 minute snooze in the afternoon! It'll make you sharper, more alert, and promote faster recuperation from intense exercise.

Herbal Approach to Better Sleep

Assuming that you're training regularly, eating five meals daily, and generally following whatever athletic lifestyle you've bought into, you shouldn't have a problem with sleep. If you do, your training methods, life's many stresses, and your diet are definitely the first areas of your lifestyle that you should scrutinize.

However, the following herbs may also be of benefit to you. The herbal blend listed at the end of this section collectively aids in calming nerves and regulating blood sugar and restorative functions, all so important in ensuring sound, beneficial sleep.

Hypnotics

Hypnotic herbs are those that can help people sleep. They do not knock people out; they just facilitate the normal, natural, sleep process. Hypnotics are herbal remedies that will help induce a deep and healing state of sleep. They have nothing at all to do with hypnotic trances!

Herbs that help you sleep have modes of action that vary from mild muscle-relaxing properties, through volatile oils that ease psychological tensions, to remedies that contain strong alkaloids that work directly on the central nervous system. Some of the most effective plant hypnotics, including opium poppy derivations, are illegal for the very degree of their effectiveness. The remedies mentioned here are entirely safe and have no addictive properties.

Hypnotic herbs should always be used within the context of approaching sleep problems through relaxation, food, and lifestyle in general. For a detailed approach to their therapeutic use, please refer to Chapter 10.

Valerian, for example, is an effective hypnotic and relaxing nervine that may be used in a whole range of stress- or anxiety-related problems. It has a calmative, an antispasmodic, and a digestive bitter effect. Valerian is also useful in the treatment of stress-related high blood pressure.

The California poppy, a common sight along any roadside in California in the spring, is a safe hypnotic and relaxing nervine that sometimes will also take the edge off pain and reduce muscle spasms.

The root of the Indian plant ashwagandha commands the same esteem for rejuvenation in Ayurvedic medicine that ginseng does in Chinese medicine. It is particularly beneficial for overworked muscles, fatigue, healing and growth of tissue, the endocrine system, sexual debility, and insomnia. It is calming and promotes deep sleep. The recommended dosage is five grams of powder twice a day in warm milk or water, sweetened with raw sugar.

Chamomile, the popular herbal tea, is taken worldwide for its soothing, relaxing effect. If you remember the story of Peter Rabbit, this was the stuff Peter's mommy brewed for him after his misadventure in Farmer MacGregor's garden. The tea is used extensively for digestive upset. To settle your stomach, steep half an ounce in one and a half cups of boiling water for 10 minutes. Drink it a few times daily as needed.

In its stronger form as an essential oil, chamomile is used for reducing fever, and as an anti-inflammatory, a burn and wound healer, a fungicide, and a sleep inducer. It is Europe's best-known cure-all. In Italy, a million cups of chamomile are consumed every day. One Italian company advertises it as a "cup of serenity."

There are plants suited to each system of the body, and some of these are hypnotics of varying strength. Despite their affinities to individual body systems, however, all hypnotic remedies can help the whole body by promoting sleep, a vital health process. See Chapter 2 for a complete discussion of these hypnotic herbs.

The rule of thumb on herbal teas is to add one teaspoon to a glass of boiling water, steep three to five minutes, and strain. Or pour the boiling water into a cup containing the herb. Add honey for taste if desired. Honey will also reduce the need to urinate during the night.

The following herbal teas are widely recommended by herbalists as soothing nightcaps:

- chamomile
- lemon balm (removes spasms and tension which might prevent sleep, can provide an energy boost if you arise tired, and is a good neural sedative; it's combined with valerian, hops, and passionflower in a German proprietary medicine to improve one's ability to fall asleep)
- passionflower (has a widespread reputation for treating sleeplessness, chronic insomnia, stress, and anxiety)
- peppermint tea (an aromatic tea with a reputation for calming, cleansing, and strengthening the entire body)
- sage (use one teaspoon of a blend combining one part sage,

one part rosemary, and two parts peppermint; add honey for enhanced calming effect)

- valerian root (may be the most effective herbal sleep inducer; used by ancient Greeks as a nerve calmer and in more modern times by the English as a tranquilizer during German air raids of World War II; helps to relieve cramps, spasms, and pain; coated capsules mask its typical bad smell)

An herbal blend to aid sleep could include:

valerian root
skullcap
hops
passionflower
royal jelly

Directions: Put 2–4 ml of the extract in warm water and drink 20 minutes before going to bed.

12

Sports Medicine in the Trenches

"Rejoice plants, bearing abundant flowers and fruit, triumphing over disease like victorious horses."

—**The Rig Veda of India**

You take chances. There is no compromise. Indeed, so long as you recognize the difference between the inherent dangers of sport and foolhardiness, risk is good. It is what gives sport its powerful allure.

Even with the most advanced training program, diet, and protective equipment, every athlete eventually must deal with injuries and illnesses, whether they're sport related or occur in the normal course of everyday life. Broken bones, torn ligaments, or concussions may be more exception than rule for most athletes, but certainly cuts, bruises, muscle soreness, and inflamed joints are ubiquitous.

Hamstring pulls are among the most common injuries athletes suffer. Groin injuries are also quite common. Furthermore, there are many injuries that are specific to certain sports. Swimming and gymnastics are notorious for shoulder injuries, for example. Many minor injuries are the result of factors including poor body mechanics, spinal imbalances, dehydration, drug use, and congenital structural weaknesses. Microtrauma brought on by training day after day without ample rest accumulates and is an often overlooked cause of injuries. Injuries, whether minor or serious, will always affect performance to some degree. For example, abrasions can be disconcerting in executing fine motor skills, and a minor muscle strain may disrupt running stride.

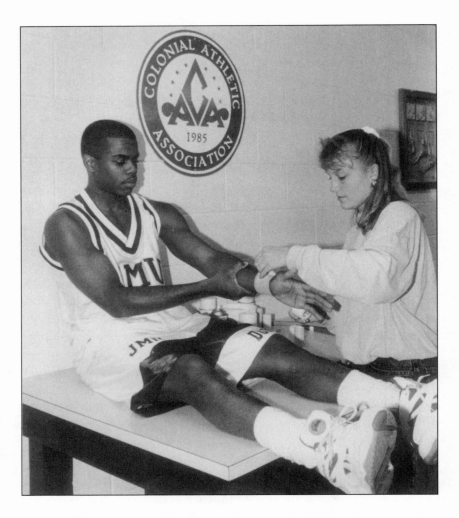

The risk of injury is omnipresent in sports. If it weren't, there would be no sport . . . only play.

While the use of herbs or other supplements cannot prevent most physical ailments, it can often help. Curative, ameliorative, and preventative herbal remedies for athletic injuries date back thousands of years. Some of these remedies help reduce pain and swelling while others have a more direct healing effect.

Before we begin, we would like to warn you that injuries, certainly major ones, will often require medical attention. *Do not assume the role of a physician!*

Arthritis

Arthritis is caused by the gradual deterioration of cartilage, usually in larger, weight-bearing joints such as the hips, knees, and spine. Cumulative microtrauma stemming from the stresses inherent in vigorous physical activity has a nasty way of becoming macrotrauma. Cartilage, not having a direct blood supply, doesn't heal as fast as other tissues. Arthritis will produce such symptoms as swelling, pain, and tenderness around affected joints.

Scientists tell us that everyone will be affected by arthritis by age 60. Some folks, especially athletes, often begin to experience arthritic symptoms as early as their twenties. There is reason to believe that athletes are especially vulnerable to arthritis. If you're a young athlete, you may not think arthritis concerns you. You feel that because of your youth, you're invincible! Do not wait until you're afflicted. Start now! Prevention, as always, is the best treatment. Who knows? Maybe you'll want to be active when you're old. Sport is not only for the young.

Some key nutritional factors in preventing arthritis include vitamins B-6, C, and E as well as manganese, selenium, and the essential fatty acids. Some herbs can be helpful as well. But by far the most effective natural treatment for arthritis is made inside your own body. It's called glucosamine.

Glucosamine

There are several types of connective tissues. Cartilage, tendons, ligaments, intervertebral discs, pads between joints, and cellular membranes all are comprised of connective tissue. All connective tissues have two common components, chief of which is collagen. One third of your body's total protein volume is comprised of collagen, making it the most common protein in the body. The other component is proteoglycan (PG), which forms the framework for collagenous tissue. These huge structural macromolecules are comprised mainly of glycosaminoglycans (GAGs)—long chains of modified sugars. The principal sugar in PG is called hyaluronic acid, of which 50 percent is comprised of glucosamine. The principal amino acids forming collagen are proline, glycine, and lysine.

Collagen and PG must somehow get together during the production of new connective tissue. Of the multitude of biochemical reactions which must take place during the synthesis of connective tissue, there is one critical rate-limiting step which, once reached, guarantees that new connective tissue is being successfully synthesized. That rate-limiting step is the conversion of glucose to glucosamine. Glucosamine, then, is the single most important substance in the synthesis of connective tissue.

More than 30 years of research has gone into understanding how glucosamine acts as the precursor of GAG synthesis. Scientists have long known that simply ingesting purified glucosamine from connective tissue allows the body to bypass the critical rate-limiting step of converting glucose to glucosamine. Here are some of the findings from these studies:

- Ninety-five percent of glucosamine is absorbed intact through the gutwall.
- Thirty percent of all orally administered glucosamine is stored for later use by the body in synthesizing more connective tissue.
- In human clinical trials, glucosamine sulfate, given orally in doses of 750 to 1,500 milligrams daily, was observed to initiate a reversal of degenerative osteoarthritis of the knee after two months. Normalization of cartilage was documented by taking biopsies of the tissue and scrutinizing them with an electron microscope.
- Of greater concern to athletes, glucosamine aids in feeding injured connective tissues, the most critical precursor for rebuilding the collagenous matrix which forms connective tissue.

- Glucosamine is the preferred substance in synthesizing PG—the framework of connective tissue.
- In vitro research demonstrated that glucosamine increases the production of GAGs (the most important molecules in PG) by 170 percent.

Glucosamine as a supplement clearly aids both in connective tissue synthesis and in the treatment of arthritis. All athletes need such a substance, as the repair and growth of connective tissue is never-ending. Glucosamine sulfate (GCS) is the only form of glucosamine you should be taking. Other products such as chondroitin sulfate, shark cartilage, and other cartilage extracts are made up of repeating molecules of glucosamine and attached sugars, and are up to 250 times larger than glucosamine sulfate. Because of the dramatic difference in size, simple GCS molecules are far more easily absorbed than chondroitin sulfate, shark cartilage, glucosamine hydrochloride, and N-acetyl-glucosamine (NAG).

Glucosamine sulfate is a simple molecule composed of glucose, an amine (nitrogen and two molecules of hydrogen), and sulfur. Your joints are rich in sulfur molecules, which form important cross-linkages with other molecules. These cross-linkages provide cartilage with its strength, structure, and shock-absorbing properties. That's yet another reason GCS is the preferred form of glucosamine.

Boswellia

Boswellia is a tree found throughout India. Its active ingredients are boswellic acids, found in the gum resin of the tree known as *salai guggul*. *Salai guggul* has been used for centuries to treat arthritis, but in present times the boswellic acids are extracted from the resin. Boswellic acids have shown no side effects in treating arthritis with doses of 400 milligrams taken three times daily.

Bromelain

Found in the stem of pineapples, bromelain contains an active ingredient known as proteolytic enzymes, which have been shown to decrease joint swelling and increase joint mobility. Recommended dosage for bromelain is between 125 and 450 milligrams taken three times daily on an empty stomach.

Capsaicin

Capsaicin is found in cayenne pepper and in many over-the-counter topical ointments. It has been shown to reduce arthritic pain in clinical studies. Some slight burning sensation may be experienced when using this ointment. Because each ointment may contain different concentrations of capsaicin, you should follow the manufacturer's directions in its use.

Devil's Claw

An ominous sounding herb, devil's claw is native to Africa and has been used for centuries in the treatment of arthritis. While many studies suggest that devil's claw will reduce pain and increase joint mobility, there are a few studies which have failed to show results. However, this may be because of poor quality of the doses used. It should not be taken during pregnancy, but up to three capsules (approximately three grams per capsule) a day is otherwise safe.

Other herbs which may be of some benefit in the treatment and prevention of arthritis include ginger, yucca saponin, and horsetail. Also see the section on inflammation later in this chapter.

Bruises

Bruises are caused by getting hit by something—a wild pitch, the helmet of a lineman, a hockey stick! Vitamin C deficiency may also be a cause. Some key nutrients in healing and preventing bruises include vitamins C, E, and K, bioflavonoids, rutin, copper, and iodine.

Arnica

An arnica compress is a long-time favorite of those who suffer from bruises. This remedy, along with speeding the healing of bruises, is also thought to work on strains and sprains. An arnica compress is easily made by combining one tablespoon arnica tincture in one pint cold water. Soak a towel in this tincture and apply it to the injured area. you can also find arnica in a sports gel form in most health food stores.

Potato

Believe it or not, a potato may help speed healing of bruises! Grate a fresh, raw potato and apply it to the bruised area. Potatoes are rich in potassium chloride, which is highly effective in healing bruises.

Cramps

Many athletes who compete in hot and humid weather conditions are particularly vulnerable to muscle cramps. There is one powerful cure for this: *water*! For whatever reason, your body does not tell you when you need water soon enough. By the time you are thirsty, dehydration has already set in. During competition, take every opportunity to drink water, even at the risk of the embarrassment of asking your coach for a time-out. Better a quick restroom break than sitting out with a painful, locked-up muscle!

Antispasmodic Tea

An effective antispasmodic tea which can help relieve and prevent muscle cramps is made by mixing one part each of: chamomile flowers, cinquefoil, lemon balm, hops, and half ounce valerian. Add one teaspoon of the herbal mixture to one cup hot water, steep three minutes, strain, and drink.

Fractures and Broken Bones

There are four classes of broken bones: simple, compound (in which the skin is broken), complicated (involving damage of internal organs), and incomplete (in which the bone is cracked but not completely broken). Unfortunately, there isn't much you can do about a broken bone; you'll have to see your doctor! But some key nutrients that can help speed recovery include calcium, vitamin A, vitamin C, and zinc. The arnica compress discussed in the section on bruises may also help.

Gotu Kola

Highly regarded as one of the most important rejuvenating herbs in Ayurvedic medicine, gotu kola has been used to promote mental calmness, fortify the immune system and adrenal glands, decrease fatigue, and strengthen bones and tendons.

Comfrey

The phytochemical alienation makes comfrey excellent for treating fractures, wounds, damaged cartilage, and muscle, and for generally speeding up the healing process. Because of its mending abilities, comfrey is also known as knitbone. It can be used as a poultice, combining it with hot water and olive oil until a thick mash is formed. Spread the mash on a linen cloth and apply to the injured area.

Inflammation

Inflammation is your body's protective response against physical blows and surgery. Your first task in treating inflammation is RICE (rest, ice, compression, and elevation). After that, there are a variety of herbs that can help reduce inflammation, as well as some key nutrients, including vitamin C, vitamin E, pantothenic acid, selenium, zinc, bioflavonoids, and fatty acids.

Chamomile

While chamomile won't cure all your ailments, it is an effective burn and wound healer, fungicide, and sleep inducer. Its most common uses are for upset stomachs and to settle the nerves, but it can also be used as an anti-inflammatory and has been known as a traditional treatment for arthritic pain and swelling. Use up to three capsules (3 grams per capsule) daily.

Bilberry

Bilberry contains a series of flavonoids known as anthocyanosides, which have strong antioxidant properties. These anthocyanosides have shown promise in reducing inflammation. You can taken up to 8 milligrams per day as an extract with an anthocyanidin content of 25 percent.

Bromelain

Found in fresh pineapple, bromelain contains proteolytic enzymes which can reduce inflammation from arthritis as well as inflammation from sports injuries. Bromelain is best taken on an empty stomach and can be consumed in doses up to 4–5 grams per day.

Curicumin

Long used in the Ayurvedic medicine practices of India, curicumin has been shown to be a more powerful anti-inflammatory than ibuprofen and as effective as cortisone. It works by stimulating the body's natural cortical steroids, increasing their half-life as well as making the receptor sites more receptive. Take four to six grams three times daily.

Devil's Claw

Please see the description of devil's claw in this chapter's section on arthritis.

Feverfew

The active component of feverfew, parthenolides, has been shown to inhibit the complex chemical process which causes inflammation and the pain resulting from it. While no long-term studies of toxicity have been conducted and no side effects documented, there are reports that chewing on the leaves of feverfew has resulted in ulcerations of the mouth as well as some swelling of the lips and tongue for some individuals. Topical solutions are available and recommended doses depend on the content of parthenolides.

Low-Back Pain

Aside from headaches, lower back pain is the leading health complaint of all people. Because of the nature of athletics, athletes are particularly susceptible to lower back pain. Perhaps the most effective prevention is to build the muscles of your lower back. Once you experience lower back pain, rest, ice, and chiropractic treatment are in order.

Some key nutrients for proper healing of lower back pain are vitamins C and D, protein, calcium, and magnesium. Two herbal remedies that can help ease lower back pain are massaging with St. John's wort oil and applying hot linseed poultice.

To prepare hot linseed poultice, soak one cup linseeds (flaxseeds) in cold water overnight, then bring to a boil. Apply as hot as tolerable.

To prepare St. John's wort oil, add fresh St. John's wort flowers to a jar and cover with olive oil. Tightly close the jar and store in warm place three to five weeks. This process will cause the oil to turn red. Strain and pour the oil into a dark-colored glass jar, and store in dark, cool area (don't refrigerate).

Burdock, chamomile, and white and black mustard may also help lower back pain. The recommended herbs in this chapter's section on inflammation may also be of benefit.

Sprains and Tendonitis

A sprain is an abnormal stretching or tearing of the ligaments that surround a joint and attach bone to bone. Ankles and knees are the most commonly sprained joints; however, you can sprain almost any ligament of the body with improper training or in a freak accident. Tendonitis, on the other hand, involves inflammation of your tendons, which attach muscle to bone.

Ample rest is needed for tendonitis, and even when it goes away, chances are it will recur sometime later. Some key nutrients for the healing of sprains and tendonitis are vitamin C, magnesium, manganese, copper, bioflavonoids, and papain. Use RICE (rest, ice, compression, and elevation) as long as swelling occurs, as well as an arnica compress for treatment. Also see this chapter's section on inflammation.

Wounds

Skin abrasions, cuts, and sores are common in everyday life, not to mention athletics! Some key nutrients involved with wound healing include B-complex vitamins, vitamin C, vitamin E, L-arginine, fatty acids, and zinc.

Aloe Vera

North and South American Indians have long valued the desert plant aloe vera for its healing abilities. Applied topically, aloe vera can promote the healing of sunburns, cuts, abrasions, wounds, and surgical incisions.

Bromelain

Already noted for its effects on inflammation, the proteolytic enzymes found in bromelain have also been shown to help in wound healing. In one particular study, 74 boxers, whose bodies were literally covered with bruises, were given 40 milligrams of bromelain four times daily for four days. Seventy-two boxers received a placebo. Seventy-eight percent of the boxers who took bromelain were bruise-free after four days and the rest within eight to ten days. Only 14 percent of those taking the placebo were as fortunate.

Recommended dosage for bromelain is between 125 and 450 milligrams taken three times daily on an empty stomach.

Tea Tree Oil

The tea tree—native to the northeast coastal region of New South Wales, Australia—contains some antiseptic properties and has been shown effective in healing a variety of skin sores when applied directly, including athlete's foot, burns, canker sores, cuts, bruises, and abrasions. It has also been used as a skin disinfectant and causes no reported irritation to the skin.

Other herbs that may promote wound healing are chamomile (applied topically), echinacea, papain, and comfrey.

Pain

"No pain, no gain."

"No guts, no glory."

"When the going gets tough, the tough get going."

Like billboards, the clichés of pain line the road to peak performance. And unless somebody up there *really* likes you, pain is indeed the price you pay for trying to excel.

Reality requires you face the music: what am I going to do about the pain that comes from gut-busting weight training for building strength, lung-bursting runs for developing endurance, and all the major and minor injuries along the way?

Be you a fitness freak, a bodybuilder, a professional athlete, or a regular weekend warrior, pain brings you to your knees. It stops your feet from taking another stride, your arms from performing another rep. It turns on the tilt light and turns off your grit.

All athletes are on a first-name basis with pain. You must learn that pain intolerance limits strength output and stymies potential. You must realize that in order to succeed you need a powerful antipain strategy. Learning to cope is not enough. You must understand what causes pain and then act to dominate it.

There are means at your disposal for combating pain and substantially increasing your pain threshold. This portion of this chapter will tell you what they are, how to use them, and in particular, educate you about the little-appreciated relationship between nutrition and pain.

What Causes Pain?

The millions of muscle cells throughout your body contract every time you call for movement. In order for this to happen, an exquisitely complex sequence of biochemical activities must take place.

Adenosine triphosphate (ATP), your body's main source of energy, is used up quickly when you start exercising. The muscle cells must create more ATP from stored creatine phosphate, then, when CP is depleted, from muscle glycogen (stored sugar). This, in turn, causes lactic acid to be produced. As it accumulates, lactic acid slows the contraction process, and oxygen is needed to convert the lactic acid back into glycogen so it may be used for energy. This biochemical sequence will continue as long as oxygen is available and you have the wherewithal to rid your muscles of toxic wastes.

Problems arise when the circulatory system cannot supply enough oxygen for the processing of lactic acid into glycogen. When this happens, lactic acid builds up and causes fatigue and attendant pain. Muscle contraction shuts down and you are thrust into metabolic turmoil wherein your heart rate as well as your breathing rate both increase by more than 100 percent. This is when you get the urge to quit and go home—not that a determined athlete like you does quit, but the urge is still there. Vince Lombardi knew about this state when he said, "Fatigue makes cowards of us all."

Your most powerful combative tool against this sort of metabolic pain is developing proper training techniques which build your tolerance to pain. These techniques must be accompanied by laser focus, tunnel vision to accomplish at all costs what your coach asks of you.

Pain from Microtrauma

Microtrauma is the result of long-term accumulation of damage done to the individual muscle cells as a result of overexertion. If allowed to continuously develop, it may cause major injuries. This microtrauma also can cause adhesions and scar tissue within the muscle that limit strength and motion.

Post-exercise muscle soreness (PEMS) is caused by this microtrauma, not lactic acid buildup, as commonly thought. While even well-conditioned athletes can get PEMS, it is most often seen in sedentary people who jump into an exercise program without reversing the effects of disuse. The sudden stress of the exercise causes minor damage to the tissues not accustomed to heavy work loads; this causes the release of an amino acid called hydroxyproline, which is one of the many that make up connective tissue. This caustic substance irritates local nerve endings and triggers pain.

To the disbelief of many people, some bodybuilders self-inflict a type of PEMS. They believe they can "shape" an individual muscle. They will "twist," "turn," "isolate," and (our favorite) "attack the muscle from different angles" in the belief that they can bypass genetics and shape a muscle. They even believe they can build muscle tissue where it doesn't exist! The "gap" between the biceps and forearm is a common example. There is no muscle tissue there, only the tendon which connects the biceps to the forearm. How big a gap you have is a matter of genetics and cannot be changed. Still, bodybuilders go on twisting, turning, isolating, and attacking, believing muscle soreness is a sign of progress!

Exertion or Weightlifter's Headache

Exercise has been known to go to your head in more ways than one. Here, we are talking about headaches caused by any type of exercise. The pain may be steady or throbbing and can last four to six hours. Some other symptoms may include blurred vision, nausea, and sweating.

Experts feel these headaches are caused by stress from the intense training which may stimulate painful dilation of blood vessels in the brain. If you have this problem, seek medical help.

Under heavy amount of weight, weightlifters have been known to clench their jaws with great pressure, often so tight they put their jaw muscles into spasm. This can produce a referred type of pain which shows up in the area of the temples. A cure? Don't clench your jaws so tight during lifts!

Supplements for Pain

The most common painkiller of all time is common aspirin, which today is a synthetic version of white willow bark. While aspirin has the advantage of low toxicity over other drugs, it can interfere with the production of muscle growth and the ability of the cells to store glucose for energy. It also increases the need for every known nutrient, including oxygen. As a result of this and for other reasons, many practitioners have started prescribing higher doses of vitamins and minerals during aspirin therapy to aid in the healing and pain-relieving process.

Vitamins and minerals are important, among other things, for energy production, immune functions, and relieving all the types of stress you place on your body. Being deficient in any vitamin or mineral will slow the healing and anti-inflammation processes and therefore prolong pain.

Vitamin C is a micronutrient which deserves extra attention for its role against pain. Studies dating back to 1966 show that vitamin C decreases lactic acid production and increases oxygen uptake by the cells, thereby reducing post-exercise soreness. It is also important for collagen, the substance which makes up connective tissue.

The daily dosage of vitamin C for pain reduction has varied from 1,000 total milligrams (taken in small and frequent doses) to as much as 10,000 milligrams! The latter recommended dosage comes from Drs. Ewan Cameron and Linus Pauling, who reported a significant pain-relief effect in patients with cancer.

A final note on vitamin C. Studies have shown that intense exercise depletes your body's stores of vitamin C. For this reason, sports nutritionists have recommended doses in the thousands of milligrams daily.

Antioxidants have been shown to have an impact on reducing pain. Strenuous exercise causes a long chain of biochemical events inside your body that contribute to free-radical formation. Free radicals are highly unstable and can damage muscle tissue, cellular membranes, and components. This chain of events can trigger muscle pains, cramps, fatigue, and other exercise-induced symptoms. Antioxidants are covered in depth in Chapter 7.

White Willow Bark

An old favorite of the ancient Egyptians, Assyrians, Greeks, and American Indians, white willow bark has been administered for a number of ailments, including headaches, fever, rheumatism, neuralgia, arthritis, gout, angina, and sore muscles.

The pain-relieving substance in white willow bark was first isolated during the 1820s, during which time salicin was isolated and identified. Later, acetylsalicylic acid was produced from salicylic acid, and thus, aspirin was born!

Yucca

Yucca has long been used by the North American Indians to reduce swelling and pain.

Ashwagandha

Ashwagandha can be considered the Ayurvedic equivalent to Chinese ginseng. It has proved to be beneficial for overworked muscles, fatigue, healing, and tissue growth.

Analgesic Balms

Analgesic balms are externally applied ointments and liniments that are rubbed over an injured area to reduce pain. They can work in many ways, including creating heat that relaxes muscles, increasing circulation, and carrying away toxins.

The Chinese have, as with many natural remedies and herbals, been forerunners in using analgesic balms for hundreds of years. Here are a few analgesic balms which you may want to try on a sprain, strain, or otherwise sore muscle or joint:

• Tiger balm contains menthol, wintergreen, eucalyptus, and lavender oil, among other ingredients. It has been known to soothe minor aches and pains, toothaches, and itching. White Flower Oil,

Kwan Loong Medicated Oil, and Temple of Heaven balm are all similar balms.

• Zheng gu shui is a powerful liniment for sprains, strains, deep bone bruises, and hairline fractures. It has been used as an anesthesia for reducing dislocations. This balm is very hot and can cause burning, blistering, and irritation to the skin. If this happens, discontinue use. It is not recommended for open wounds or for fair-skinned people.

• Tieh ta yao gin is quite similar to zheng gu shui, but is less powerful. Still, it is good for minor sprains and contusions.

• Chinese muscle oil can be used to treat tight muscles and other injuries. It is especially effective when applied before and after stretching.

Illness and Health

What is health and what makes a person healthy? Health textbooks, doctors, coaches, athletes, laypeople have all tried their hand at defining *health.* Many textbooks have listed a simple definition of health as "the absence of illness" or "freedom from disease." True, being ill certainly means there is something wrong with your health, but you can sit in your easy chair for days and not be ill. Does that mean you are healthy? No, of course not. So, look at the word *disease* or *dis-ease* as meaning "not at ease." A related, and perhaps more personal, definition may be "your ability to meet the normal exigencies of your lifestyle with ease, and still have the ability to cope with life's little emergencies."

OK, now we're getting somewhere! To be healthy, you must not be ill and your energy reserves must be high enough to meet both your lifestyle requirements and minor emergencies head-on. But what about your mental capacity and your emotional and social health? The World Health Organization (WHO) has addressed these problems in its definition: "Health is more than simply the absence of illness. It is the active state of physical, emotional, mental, and social well-being."

There's nothing new about this definition. Actually, around the turn of the century, the YMCA purloined a symbol from American Indian culture which is very close to this definition. Their famous triangle logo signifies the interrelatedness of body, mind, and spirit.

Moderation in Exercise

"Moderation is the key to healthful living." This statement has been echoed by some of the greatest philosophers, doctors, and healers throughout the ages. Is it true that too much of something, even if it's good for you, can hurt you?

What about exercise? Can you exercise too much? Yes! You cannot continue exercising at high levels and expect to stay healthy. Running, weightlifting, aerobics, and all other forms of exercise in excess can lower the immune system. Take the viewpoints of Ron Lawrence, M.D., past president of the American Medical Athletic Association. Lawrence, who has run more than 150 marathons himself, believes "Exercise done at a non-exhausting level enhances the immune system. . . . Too much [exercise] and [the immune system] depletes."

Lawrence claims that a marathon runner's immune system after long-distance races may be lowered severely for many weeks after the race. He has seen many people "get sick as hell with anything from hepatitis to the common cold after exhaustive training or races." He further submits, "I haven't personally experienced this same susceptibility—or seen it among others—after 10 kilometer races or less stressful events."

These statements are backed with solid data. In a study of more than 2,000 runners who competed in the 1987 Los Angeles marathon and those who trained but didn't compete, it was found that within a week after the race 13 percent of the competing runners reported a cold, flu, or sore throat. Only 2 percent of the trained runners who didn't compete reported similar symptoms. These results led researchers to the conclusion that running more than 60 miles per week doubles the odds of infection or sickness as compared to running 20 miles or less per week. Furthermore, injuries to your hips, knees, ankles, and shins are more likely with running excessive miles in a short time period.

Similar results have been seen in cross-country skiers as well as weightlifters. Lawrence reports that many weightlifters who engage in training with extremely high levels of intensity often experience colds and infections as well. This may be compounded with the use of anabolic steroids (a practice still all-too widespread among athletes of all sports persuasions) which can further lower the effectiveness of your immune system.

Moderation is definitely an important part of constructing your training program. But if you are a marathon runner, weightlifter or any other athlete, you *must* train hard before a competition. This creates a difficult situation, as the training and even the competition itself take their toll on your immune system. There are two things you can do to reduce your chances of becoming ill: (1) periodize your program and (2) supplement your diet.

At this point, you should go back to Chapter 3 to review the fundamentals of establishing a periodized training program and nutritional protocol for your sport. You will note that proper nutrition and supplementation can have a tremendous effect on your immune system's competence regardless of where you are in your yearly training cycle. Many vitamins and minerals are needed for your immune system's health and integrity. Several herbs have been shown to have immune-boosting properties. Taking these herbs not only in times of heavy training but year-round can help your immune system work at optimal levels.

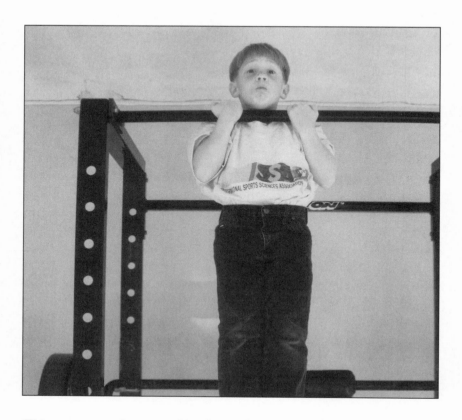

This young man has everything he needs—now—to be a great athlete someday.

Glossary of Herbal and Nutrition Terms

acetyl coenzyme A—A chief precursor of lipids, it is formed by an acetyl group attaching itself to coenzyme A (CoA) during the oxidation of amino acids, fatty acids, or pyruvate.

acidophilus (*lactobacillus acidophilus*)—The "friendly" bacteria (also called intestinal flora) our body needs to have an ideal digestive process. Frequently the colon may lack these indispensable bacteria because of the intake of antibiotics, corticosteroids, sugar, and yeast, or because of stress. The end result is often growth of yeast (*candida albicans*).

adaptogens—Agents that help the body cope with stress through biochemical support of the adrenal glands. Term was coined by researchers to describe the action of a substance that helps increase resistance to adverse physical and environmental influences. To be a true adaptogen the substance must (1) be safe for daily use, (2) increase the body's resistance to a wide variety of factors, and (3) have a normalizing action in the body. Adaptogens can help otherwise healthy individuals adapt to stresses such as increased work load, illness, or injury.

additives—Substances other than foodstuff present in food as a result of production, processing, storage, or packaging. Examples include preservatives, coloring, thickeners (gums), excipients, and binders.

albumin—Type of simple protein widely distributed throughout the tissues and fluids of plants and animals. Varieties of albumin are found in blood, milk, egg white, wheat, barley, and muscle.

alfalfa (*medicago sativa*)—Plant that is 25 percent protein by weight and contains eight important enzymes that enhance food assimilation. It is also rich in many other nutrients, including vitamin B-6, an essential co-factor in the body's metabolism of muscle-building protein.

aloe vera (*aloe barbandenis*)—Desert plant long valued by North and South American Indians for its healing abilities. Applied topically, aloe vera can promote the healing of sunburns, cuts, abrasions, wounds, and surgical incisions.

alpha ketoisocaproate (KIC)—An alpha-ketoacid of L-leucine. It is well supported in research literature as a stimulant of lymphocyte blastogenesis and antibody response, and it can also increase muscle growth and decrease fat deposits. Recently, KIC has been used extensively in fat-loss preparations and in high protein supplements used clinically to retard muscle-wasting.

alteratives—Agents that work by gradually restoring proper body functioning. One main function of alteratives is neutralizing toxins in the blood. Also called "blood cleansers," but because alteratives help the kidneys, liver, lungs, skin, and other systems remove toxins, the term is not complete.

althea root marshmallow, or hollyhock (*Althaea officinalis*)—Marshmallow is one of the more popular demulcents. The leaf is used to treat bronchitis and other forms of respiratory distress as well as urinary problems. The root is used to treat digestive-system problems such as gastritis, gastric or peptic ulceration, ulcerative colitis, enteritis, and inflammation of the mouth or pharynx.

amino acids—The building blocks of protein. There are 24 amino acids, which form countless different proteins. All contain nitrogen, oxygen, carbon, and hydrogen. Amino acids are either essential or nonessential. The eight essential aminos must be derived from food. They are: L-isoleucine, L-leucine, L-lysine, L-methionine, L-phenylalanine, L-tryptophan, L-threonine, and L-valine. Two others, L-arginine and L-histidine, are essential for children. Nonessential aminos are manufactured internally in the quantities the body requires. They are: L-alanine, L-asparagine, L-aspartic acid, L-citrulline, L-cysteine, L-cystine, L-glutamine, L-glutamic acid, glycine, L-ornithine, L-proline, L-serine, taurine, and L-tyrosine.

ammonia scavengers—A toxic by-product of intense training caused by the breakdown of amino acids for energy. Ammonia can accumulate to cause severe fatigue. Combinations of certain amino acids and minerals (especially glutamic acid in combination with vitamin B-6) help remove ammonia from the blood.

angelica (*Angelica archangelica*)—Herb with a reputation for being a powerful carminative, soothing an upset stomach, and improving gastrointestinal function. More recently, it has been used to aid those suffering from anorexia. When combined with other herbs, angelica has been shown to have anticancer properties.

anticatarrhals—Substances that help your body get rid of excess mucous from the lungs, sinuses, and throat.

anti-inflammatories—Substances that reduce swelling and pain in various bodily tissues. Most herbs with anti-inflammatory properties contain volatile oils and work by relaxing the nervous system and muscle spasms, attacking bacteria, or increasing blood flow to the affected area.

antimicrobials or antibacterials—Substances that stimulate the immune system, or directly attack micro-organisms and bacteria to keep them from disrupting the body's systems and causing illness.

antispasmodics—Medicines that relieve muscle cramps by alleviating muscular tension, nervous tension, or psychological tension.

antioxidants—Substances such as vitamins, minerals, and phytochemicals that protect against free radicals. Free-radical scavengers (another term for antioxidants) include vitamins A, C, and E, glutathione, selenium, zinc, and many phytochemicals such as the proanthocyanadins and nordihydroguairetic acid. *See* **free radicals**.

antispasmodic tea—An effective antispasmodic tea which can help relieve and prevent muscle cramps. Made by mixing one part each of chamomile flowers, cinquefoil, lemon balm, hops, and half ounce valerian. Add one teaspoon herbal mixture to one cup hot water, steep three minutes, strain, and drink.

arachidonic acid—An essential fatty acid found in the liver, brain, and other organs. It is the biosynthetic precursor of prostaglandins. In experiments with mice, the deprivation of all fat intake caused scaly skin, kidney lesions, bloody urine, and early death. These conditions were cured by the administration of arachidonic acid, linoleic acid, and linolenic acid. Arachidonic acid is used therapeutically as a nutrient.

arnica (*Arnica montana*)—Remedy that speeds healing of bruises and is thought to work on strains and sprains. To make an arnica compress, combine one tablespoon arnica tincture in one pint cold water. Soak a towel in this mixture and apply to the injured area.

ashwagandha (*Withania somnifera*)—Herb that has proved to be beneficial for overworked muscles, fatigue, healing, and tissue growth. Also known as Indian ginseng, it has been clinically shown to be useful as a remedy for anxiety and has been used as an adaptogenic.

astragalus (*Astragalus membranaceus*)—Herb that is particularly useful for athletes who suffer from shortness of breath. It increases endurance, helps protect adrenal function, and promotes the efficiency of the immune system. The active ingredients in astragalus are an isoflavone known as 4 'hydroxy-3'-methoxyisoflavone 7-sug, triterpenoid saponins, and numerous polysaccharides shown to enhance the immune system.

astringents—Substances that tighten or bond tissues together by binding protein molecules, causing contraction and firming of tissues. Useful for cuts, abrasions, sinusitis, and diarrhea.

balm (*Melissa officinalis*)—Plant containing a phytochemical called chrysin that has been clinically shown to increase luteinizing hormone (LH), a hormone produced in the pituitary gland that is responsible for regulating testosterone production. Theoretically, increasing LH indirectly increases testosterone. There is also evidence that chrysin can block cortisol, the body's natural catabolic agent, thus dramatically increasing anabolic processes, which are spurred by the presence of testosterone.

bergamot (*Citrus bergamia*)—Herb that may be useful in relieving hypotension, as well as symptoms of the common cold.

beta carotene—A carotenoid (pigment) found in yellow, orange, and deep green vegetables, which provides a source of vitamin A when ingested. This substance has been found to have antioxidant and anticancer properties.

bilberry (*Vaccinium myrtillus*)—Plant containing anthocyanosides. Folklore and studies show bilberry extract protects blood capillaries and the heart, is an excellent anti-inflammatory, and inhibits cholesterol-induced atherosclerosis and clotting.

bioflavonoids (vitamin P)—Water-soluble substances that appear in fruits and vegetables as companions to vitamin C. They are: citrin, rutin, hesperidin, flavone, and flavonols. They increase the strength of capillaries and regulate their permeability for the countless biochemical transfers that occur between blood and tissue. No RDA. Dietary sources include citrus fruit pulp, apricots, buckwheat, and berries.

biotin—A member of the B-complex vitamin family and essential for metabolism of fat, protein, and vitamins C and B-12. It helps alleviate muscle pains, eczema, dermatitis. No RDA. Dietary sources include egg yolk, liver, whole rice, and brewer's yeast.

bitters—Classification of herbs that help the body detoxify itself. The bitter sensation triggers a hormonal response in the digestive system, which leads to the production of digestive juices and bile, and detoxifies the liver. Bitters can also stimulate intestinal healing.

black cohosh (*Cimicifuga racemosa*)—Herb used for centuries by American Indians. Black cohosh may be useful in relieving swelling and pain from rheumatism. Clinically, black cohosh has been shown to relieve menopause symptoms.

black mustard (*Brassica nigra*)—Commonly known to be stronger than white mustard, black mustard can be used to soothe joint pain.

blue vervian (*Verbena hastada*)—Herb commonly used as a natural tranquilizer. The antiperiodic properties of its root stock and leaves relieve nervous tension and make it an excellent sleep aid.

borage (*Borago officinalis*)—Contains gamma linolenic acid (GLA), which helps the body convert linoleic acid into prostaglandin E1—a conversion easily blocked by outside sources including viruses, cholesterol, and alcohol. Allowing this conversion to take place decreases blood cholesterol levels and lowers blood pressure.

boron—A nonmetallic earth element. It is required by some plants as a trace element and occurs as a hard crystalline solid or as brown powder. Boron forms compounds such as boric acid or borax. Taken as a supplement boron has been shown to combat osteoporosis in middle-aged women. Despite widespread use as a bodybuilding supplement, there is no evidence that it has anabolic properties.

boswellin (*Boswellia serrata*)—Herb containing boswellic acids found in the gum resin of the *salai guggul* tree, used for centuries to treat arthritis.

brahmi (*Centella asiatica*)—*See* **gotu kola.**

branched-chain amino acids (BCAA)—The amino acids L-leucine, L-isoleucine, and L-valine, which have a particular molecular structure that gives them their name. The BCAAs comprise 35 percent of muscle tissue and, particularly L-leucine, help increase work capacity by stimulating production of insulin, the hormone that opens muscle cells to glucose. BCAAs are burned as fuel during highly intense training and at the end of long-distance events when the body recruits protein for as much as 20 percent of its energy needs.

brewer's yeast (*Saccharomyces cerevisiae*)—A nonleavening yeast used as a nutritional supplement for its rich content of vitamins (particularly B complex), minerals, and amino acids.

brindall berry—Plant containing hydroxycitric acid (HCA) which is cited in research as able to inhibit fat synthesis.

bromelain—Found in the stem of pineapples, this substance contains an active ingredient known as proteolytic enzymes, which have been shown to decrease joint swelling and increase joint mobility.

burdock (*Arcticum lappa*)—Traditionally used as a blood purifier as well as a treatment for joint pain. Burdock also contains inulin, which has been clinically shown to be useful in controlling blood sugar.

caffeine—A chemical (a methyl derivative of xanthine), occurring in coffee, black tea, and cola drinks, that can stimulate the nervous system. In small amounts, it can create mental alertness. In larger amounts, it can cause nervousness, anxiety, and sleeplessness and is used medicinally as a diuretic and headache remedy. It has also been known to stimulate the central nervous system, mobilize various hormones and tissue substrates involved in metabolic processes, improve muscle contraction, and improve mobilization and utilization rates of fats and carbohydrates for energy.

calcium—The most abundant mineral in the body, a vital factor for bones, teeth, muscle growth, muscle contraction, the regulation of nutrient passage in and out of cells, and nerve transmissions. RDA is 800 to 1,400 milligrams; dose increases with age. Dietary sources include milk and dairy products, soybeans, sardines, salmon, peanuts, beans, and green vegetables.

calmatives and carminatives—Substances containing aromatic volatile oils that reduce inflammation in the intestinal walls, promoting proper functioning of the digestive system, relieving intestinal pain, and removing gas. Calmatives' effects on the digestive system will promote better nutrient absorption and help relieve upset stomach. Like calmatives, carminatives have strong effects on the digestive system. They ease gas, indigestion, and intestinal cramping and can also stimulate your appetite.

capsaicin—*See* **cayenne**.

capsicum—*See* **cayenne**.

caraway (*Carum carvi*)—Herb containing the phenolic compound capsaicin, which has a well-demonstrated effect in lowering blood cholesterol levels. It has also been used as a digestive aid and to reduce nausea.

carbohydrate—Chemical compound of carbon, oxygen, and hydrogen, usually with hydrogen and oxygen in the right proportions to form water. Common forms are starches, sugars, cellulose, dextrins, glycogen, and gums. One of the three basic foodstuffs, carbohydrates are more readily used for energy production than are fats and proteins and can be classified as either simple or complex.

cardamom (*Elettaria cardomomum*)—Herb that acts as a digestive stimulant as well as a blood thinner.

cayenne (*Capsicum frutescens*)—Herb used as a general stimulant for the gastrointestinal and cardiovascular systems. As an appetite stimulant, it increases the flow of saliva and other digestive juices and increases the rate and efficiency of nutrient absorption. Cayenne contains the phenolic compound capsaicin or capsicum, which has a demonstrated effect in lowering blood cholesterol levels.

chamomile (*Matricaria chamomilla*)—Herb known in Europe as a "cure-all," it is an effective burn and wound healer, fungicide, and sleep inducer. Its most common uses are for upset stomachs and to settle the nerves, but it can also be used as an anti-inflammatory and it has been known as a traditional treatment for arthritic pain and swelling.

chaparral (*Larrea tridentata*)—Plant containing an antioxidant phytochemical called nordihydroguaiaretic acid (NGDA), which may help ward off infections, cancerous tumors, and cellular damage resulting from free-radical activity.

Chinese muscle oil—Herbal that can be used to treat tight muscles and other injuries. It is especially effective when applied before and after stretching.

choline—A B-complex vitamin associated with utilization of fats and cholesterol in the body, and a constituent of lecithin, which helps prevent fats from building up in the liver and blood. It is essential for the health of myelin sheath, a principal component of nervous tissue, and plays an important role in transmission of nerve impulses. No RDA. Dietary sources include lecithin, egg yolk, liver, and wheat germ.

chromium—Along with niacin, an essential micronutrient that activates insulin for vital functions relating to blood sugar, muscle growth, and energy. It also helps control cholesterol. Chromium deficiency is widespread as a result of depletion caused by exercise and high sugar consumption. No RDA. Dietary sources include brewer's yeast, shellfish, chicken liver, and oysters. Commercially available chromium supplements include picolinate (chromium bound to zinc) and polynicotinate (chromium bound to niacin) varieties. Research is unclear as to their respective anabolic activities, but both appear to enhance the activity of glucose-tolerance-factor (GTF) regulators. That is, they aid in regulating blood sugar, and therefore insulin, levels.

ciwujia (*Radix acanthopanax senticosus*)—Herb used in China for more than 1,700 years and recently clinically shown to prevent or treat fatigue, increase endurance, and boost the immune system.

clove (*Eugenia caryophyllata*)—Herb with antimicrobial properties. Antimicrobials help ward off infections by eliminating the pathogen or by boosting the body's immune system.

colostrum—The first lacteral secretions obtained after paturition; the conclusion of pregnancy. Powerful growth factors and immune modulators are provided the newborn infant through this medium, particularly during the first few days after birth. Used as a supplement among adults, colostrum is a well-known provider of antiviral, antibacterial, antifungal, and antiallergenic properties.

comfrey (*Symphytum officinale*)—Plant with phytochemical allantoin that aids in treating fractures, wounds, damaged cartilage and muscle, and generally speeding up the healing process. Because of its mending abilities, comfrey is also known as "knitbone."

complete protein—Refers to protein which contains all essential amino acids in sufficient quantity and in the right ratio to maintain a positive nitrogen balance. The egg is the most complete protein food in nature, with an assimilability ratio of 94 to 96 percent. That is, up to 96 percent of the protein in eggs will be used as protein. In contrast, only about 60 to 70 percent of the protein in milk, meat, or fish can be used as protein. *See* **essential amino acids**.

complex carbohydrates—Foods of plant origin consisting of three or more simple sugars bound together. Also known as polysaccharides. The starch in grains is an example. Compared to monosaccharides (refined carbohydrates such as table sugar and white-flour products), complex carbs require a prolonged enzymatic process for digestion and thus provide a slow, even, and ideal flow of energy. This avoids fluctuations in glucose (blood sugar) levels, which can affect energy. Complex carbs contain fiber and many nutrients.

copper—Mineral that helps convert the body's iron into hemoglobin for oxygen transportation through the bloodstream. Essential for utilization of vitamin C. No RDA. Dietary sources include legumes, whole wheat, prunes, liver, and seafood.

cornsilk (*Zea mays*)—Plant containing saponins and alkaloids which are useful as diuretics, demulcents, and anti-inflammatories. May be useful in treating urinary infections such as cystitis, urethritis, and prostatitis.

couch grass (*Agropyron repens*)—Plant with rhizome that is used as a diuretic, demulcent, and anti-inflammatory. Couch grass is often used for urinary infections, to soothe irritation and inflammation, for kidney stones, and for the treatment of enlarged prostate glands. It is also used with other herbs for the treatment of rheumatism.

creatine monohydrate—Substance clinically shown to improve plasma creatine concentrations in muscle cells by as much as 50 percent. Research shows this substance to be effective in improving training intensity and recovery. It is able to pass through the gut wall and into the bloodstream intact, and upon entering the muscle cells, is converted into creatine phosphate (CP). *See* **creatine phosphate**.

creatine phosphate (CP)—Organic compound in muscle fibers that is fractured enzymatically for the production of ATP, the body's basic fuel that generates muscle contractions.

cumin (*Cuminum cyminu*)—Carminative that has a strong effect on the digestive system. It can be used to ease gas, indigestion, intestinal cramping, and also to stimulate your appetite.

curicumin—The yellow pigment of tumeric. Curicumin has been shown to be a more powerful anti-inflammatory than ibuprofen and as effective as cortisone. It works by stimulating the body's natural cortical steroids, increasing their half-life as well as making the receptor cites more receptive.

cypress (*Cupressus*)—Plant that has been used to strengthen blood vessels. It can also be useful in treating laryngitis.

damiana leaf (*Turnera diffusa*)—Plant with volatile oils and flavonoids that can be used as a nerve tonic, antidepressant, urinary antiseptic, and laxative.

dandelion (*Taraxacum officinale*)—Plant used to promote the liver's production of bile, the fluid secreted into the small intestine to break down dietary fat. Dandelions are also effective as diuretics, as mild laxatives, for treatment of fungus infections, for enhancing adrenal function, and to help prevent anemia by strengthening the blood. There is also evidence that one phytochemical in dandelions, inulin, may be beneficial to diabetics. The greens, flowers, and root juices are all beneficial.

dehydroepiandrosterone (DHEA)—Ruled a hormone by the FDA, DHEA is the second most abundant steroid molecule in humans. The ruling is controversial because, whereas hormones tend to be held in reserve in the gland which produced them and liberated as needed, DHEA is produced by the adrenal gland and immediately released into the bloodstream for cellular metabolism. Research tends to support its anti-obesity, anti-aging, energizing, memory-enhancing, immune boosting, cardiotonic, and anticarcinogenic activities. It is widely available as a nutritional supplement and appears to have few side effects, most notably mild androgenic activity. DHEA is banned by virtually all sport governing bodies.

demulcents—Agents that have an anti-inflammatory and soothing effect on the kidneys, bladder, and mucous membranes, and can help avoid compromising proper waste elimination. They also help moisten these tissues. Demulcents can also ease inflammation, dryness, and irritation of the mucous membranes found in the throat and nasal cavity.

devil's claw (*Harpagophytum procumbens*)—Herb clinically shown to reduce pain and increase joint mobility.

diaphoretics—Agents that cause perspiration, thus eliminating toxins through the skin. By dilating capillaries near the skin's surface—which also improves overall blood circulation—or relaxing pores, diaphoretics help toxins more easily pass into sweat glands where they are discarded. Diaphoretics also support kidney function, where toxins are separated from the blood and discarded in the urine.

diuretics—Agents that increase production and removal of urine, thus eliminating toxins and waste from the body. Ancient herbal tradition has it that diuretics include any herb beneficial to the urinary system's overall health. Many herbs, including parsley root, uva ursi, cornsilk, alfalfa, juniper berries, artichokes, asparagus, astragalus, buchu, burdock, celery, chaparral, dandelion, kava kava, and sarsaparilla are known to have diuretic properties. Diuretics should not be used long-term and definitely not during intense exercise as they can rob the body of minerals and fluids that are vital during exercise.

dL-phenylalanine (**DLPA**)—A mixture consisting of equal parts of the D- and L-forms of phenylalanine. Phenylalanine is a naturally occurring amino acid, discovered in 1879, essential for optimal growth in infants and for nitrogen equilibrium in human adults. DLPA is used in the control of pain through a mechanism believed to involve a sparing effect on opiatelike substances naturally secreted by the brain (i.e., endorphins and enkephalins).

echinacea (*Echinacea angustifolia*)—Herb found to stimulate white blood cells that destroy micro-organisms such as bacteria and viruses. It also inhibits the activity of an enzyme which erodes intracellular tissue and permits pathogens to weaken the body.

eicosapentaenoic acid (**EPA**)—Fatty acid found in fish and fish oils, which is believed to lower cholesterol, especially cholesterol bound to low density lipoproteins (**LDL**).

electrolytes—Minerals such as sodium, potassium, chloride, calcium, and magnesium that provide conductivity functions for fluid passage through cellular membranes.

enzymes—Chemical ferment proteins secreted by or contained within cells, which act as catalysts to induce chemical changes in other substances without being changed themselves. Enzymes are specific in their actions, acting only on specific substances called substrates. They are present in the digestive fluids and in many of the tissues, and are capable of producing in small amount the transformation on a large scale of various compounds. They are divided into six main groups: oxidoreductases, transferases, hydrolases, lyases, isomerases, and ligases.

ergogens—Aids that comprise a host of substances or treatments that may improve physiological performance or remove psychological barriers associated with more intense activity. They can be nutritional, physiological, psychological, mechanical, physical, environmental, or pharmacological in nature.

essential amino acids—Those amino acids that the body cannot make for itself. They are: isoleucine, leucine, lysine, methionine, phenylalanine, tryptophan, and valine.

essential fatty acids—Acids that aid in oxygen transport through blood to all cells, tissues, and organs, help maintain resilience and lubrication of all cells, and combine with protein and cholesterol to form living membranes that hold body cells together. They break up cholesterol deposits on arterial walls, thereby preventing arteriosclerosis. Fatty acids are necessary for the function of the thyroid and adrenal glands. Three are referred to as essential fatty acids because they are vital for sustaining optimal health. They are: linoleic acid, linolenic acid, and arachidonic acid.

eucalyptus (*Eucalyptus globulus*)—Herb mainly comprised of volatile oils that can help ward off infections, ease muscle cramps and tension, and act as a stimulant. It also can work as an expectorant to help remove excess mucous from the lungs.

evening primrose oil (EPO) (*Oenothera biennis*)—Oil containing high amounts of an essential fatty acid known to prevent hardening of the arteries, heart disease, and high blood pressure. It is known to reduce cholesterol and inflammation, protect the liver, and improve pancreatic function.

expectorants—Herbs that remove phlegm and excess fluid from the lungs as well as the throat. Expectorants are also useful for bronchitis and ashram.

fat—Chemical compounds that are not as readily converted to energy as are carbohydrates. Saturated fatty acids are generally solid at room temperature and are derived primarily from animal sources. Unsaturated fatty acids are usually liquid and come from vegetable, nut, or seed sources. The body's fat deposits surround and protect organs such as the kidneys, heart, and liver. Subcutaneous fat insulates the body from environmental temperature changes, thereby preserving body heat.

fat (total)—Term describing the fat consumed from both saturated and unsaturated sources. High total dietary fat intake increases risk of obesity, some types of cancer, and possibly gallbladder disease.

fat-soluble vitamins—Vitamins which can be dissolved in fats or fatty tissue. They are: vitamins A, D, E, and K.

fatty acid—One of the building blocks of fat. Used as fuel for muscle contractions. Fatty acids aid in oxygen transport through blood to all cells, tissues, and organs. They help maintain resilience and lubrication of all cells, and combine with protein and cholesterol to form living membranes that hold body cells together. They break up cholesterol deposits on arterial walls, thereby preventing arteriosclerosis. Fatty acids are necessary for the function of the thyroid and adrenal glands. *See* **essential fatty acids**.

fennel (*Foeniculum vulgare*)—Herb containing aromatic volatile oils which reduce inflammation in the intestinal walls, promoting proper functioning of the digestive system as well as relieving intestinal pain and removing gas. As a calmative, fennel's effects on the digestive system promote better absorption of nutrients and help relieve upset. It can also be used to relieve painful, stiff joints.

fenugreek (*Trigonella foenum-graecum*)—Herb containing the phenolic compound capsaicin, which has a well-demonstrated effect in lowering blood cholesterol levels. Research suggests fenugreek may help regulate blood sugar and may be useful for diabetics. Historically it has been used as a remedy for sore throats.

feverfew (*Tanacetum parthenium*)—Herb containing the active component parthenolides which have been shown to inhibit the complex chemical process that causes inflammation and the pain resulting from it.

fiber (dietary)—The indigestible complex carbohydrates that make up plant cell walls. They include cellulose, hemicellulose, pectin, and a variety of gums, mucilages, and algal polysaccharides. Healthy intestines and regular elimination require adequate fiber. A diet low in fiber is associated with constipation, intestinal disorders, varicose veins, obesity, and heart disease.

flaxseed (*Linnum usitatissimum*)—A demulcent which can help soothe and protect the tissues of the digestive system. Complex polysaccharides in flaxseed are the main phytochemicals involved in this process.

folic acid—A B-complex vitamin essential in formation of red blood cells and metabolism of protein. Important for proper brain function, mental and emotional health, appetite, and production of hydrochloric acid. It is very often deficient in diets. RDA is 400 micrograms. Dietary sources include green leafy vegetables, liver, and brewer's yeast.

gamma oryzanol—A substance extracted from rice bran oil which some athletes believe has nonsteroidal, growth-promoting properties when taken as a supplement. It allegedly helps increase lean body mass and strength, decreases fatty tissue, improves recovery from workouts, and reduces post-workout muscle soreness, particularly among female athletes. Recently, in preliminary testing, its active ingredient, ferulic acid, was reported to exert an even more pronounced effect than gamma oryzanol.

garlic (*Allium sativum*)—Herb with an international reputation as a remedy that lowers blood pressure and generally improves the health of the cardiovascular system. A recent study led clinicians to conclude that the essential oil of garlic possessed a distinct fat-reducing action in both healthy people and patients with coronary heart disease. Garlic contains allicin, a thiosulfinate which is thought to reduce the tendency for unnecessary clotting within blood vessels. Traditional use of garlic in the treatment of hypertension is only sparsely supported by research.

gentian root (*Gentiana lutea*)—One of the strongest bitters known. It has proved to be an excellent treatment against several forms of digestive disease, including dyspepsia. Gentian root has also been clinically shown to stimulate the digestive system to secrete digestive juices for faster, more complete food digestion, absorption, and assimilation.

geranium (*Geranium sanguineum*)—The antiviral action of a polyphenolic complex isolated from the medicinal plant *Geranium sanguineum* showed a positive effect on inhibiting the reproduction of herpes simplex virus type 1 as well as an anti-influenza action. Central nervous system depressive and hypotensive actions of other geranium phytochemicals were also noted in other studies.

germanium—A trace mineral (number 32 on the periodic table), it has been tested and used for the treatment of a variety of medical problems that require improved oxygenation and immune function, ranging from simple viral infections to cancer. It is found in the soil, in foods, and in many plants such as aloe vera, garlic, and ginseng.

gilead (*Populus candicans*)—Herb containing a phytochemical called chrysin which has been clinically shown to increase luteinizing hormone (LH), the hormone responsible for regulating testosterone production. *See* **balm**.

ginger (*Zingiber officinale*)—Herb containing aromatic essential oils, antioxidants, and the pungent oleoresins historically used for treating motion sickness and nausea, improving capillary permeability, reducing cholesterol absorption in the gut, reducing inflammation, and improving cardiovascular functioning. As a carminative, ginger has a strong effect on the digestive system. It can be used to ease gas, indigestion, and intestinal cramping and can also stimulate the appetite.

ginger root (*Zingiber officinale*)—Herb used as a stimulant of the circulatory system, carminative, anti-spasmodic, rubefacient, and diaphoretic.

ginkgo biloba—Plant containing quercetin and flavoglycosides as its active components. Ginkgo extract is shown to (1) reduce clots or thrombi formation in the veins and arteries, (2) increase cellular energy by increasing cellular glucose and ATP,(3) scavenge free radicals, (4) prevent formation of free radicals, (5) reduce high blood pressure, and (6) promote peripheral blood flow, especially to the brain, and (7) ameliorate inner ear problems. Ginkgo also has been shown to improve alertness, short-term memory, and various other cognitive disorders.

ginseng—Some of the best-known adaptogens are among the over 200 varieties of ginsengs. American ginseng (*panax quiquinfolia*) and the Oriental ones, the most common of which is *panax ginseng*, are two examples of widely used adaptogens. The word *panax* is derived from the latin *panacea*, meaning "cure-all." (*See* **adaptogens**.)

glucosamine—The most important substance in the synthesis of connective tissues, which include: cartilage, tendons, ligaments, intervertebral discs, pads between joints, and cellular membranes. It is available as a popular supplement in the form of glucosamine sulfate.

glucagon—A hormone secreted by the alpha cells of the pancreas, which stimulates the breakdown of glycogen and the release of glucose by the liver, thereby causing an increase in blood sugar levels. It works in direct opposition to insulin. Liver glucose is freed when the blood-sugar level drops to around 70 milligrams/100 milligrams of blood. Exercise and starvation both increase glucagon levels, as does the presence of amino acids in the blood after a high-protein meal. Glucagon produces a smooth muscle relaxation when administered parenterally.

glucose polymers—A low glycemic carbohydrate supplement that delivers a steady source of energy for workouts and restoration. Branching glucose polymers (i.e., glucose molecules comprised of differing glycemic indexes due to their structural complexity) are available as drinks, powders, and tablets.

goathead (*Tribulus terrestris*)—Herb that has become widely popular in the bodybuilding community for its ability to increase production of luteinizing hormone directly as opposed to increasing it indirectly via anti-estrogen activity. Theoretically, increasing LH also increases testosterone production. Goathead has also been used for centuries in various parts of the world to treat infertility and impotence.

goldenseal (*Hydrastis canadensis*)—Herb containing alkaloids, especially berberine, that make it useful as an immune system stimulant.

gotu kola (*Centella asiatica*)—The primary Indian remedy for nervous conditions, insomnia, stress, and disturbed emotions. Gotu kola is popular for promoting mental calm and clear thinking and also for fortifying the immune system and adrenal glands. In China it is a frequent prescription for regeneration and is widely used to enhance memory, decrease fatigue, nourish the blood, strengthen bones and tendons, and calm nerves.

green tea—Plant also known as GTA (green tea antioxidant) or GTE (green tea extract). It has been clinically shown to be as much as 200 times more effective than vitamin E at scavenging hydrogen peroxide and superoxide anion radicals. *See* **free radicals**. As such, it is perhaps the most potent antioxidant known to man in its ability to prevent antibacterial and antiviral activity, antiplatelet and hypocholesterolemic activity, lung cancer due to smoking, skin damage and skin cancer due to radiation, and a host of other age-related maladies. The active ingredients of green tea are called polyphenol catechins. Green tea is unprocessed; black tea is the same plant but highly processed tea. Oolong tea, also from the same plant, is partially processed.

gymnema sylvestre—An Indian Ayurvedic medicine that has been used in India for diabetes, and snakebites and as a diuretic, stomachic, and urinary antiseptic.

hawthorn berries (*Crataegus oxycantha*)—Plant containing flavonoids that have been shown to dilate blood vessels, which helps alleviate hypertension and high blood pressure. Hawthorn berries are an excellent cardiovascular tonic and also contain procyanidins, which act as a sedative and antispasmodic.

hepatics—Substances that aid liver function. The liver is an important organ for many reasons including waste removal. Hepatics can help the liver eliminate excess ammonia and lactic acid that can build up during exercise.

herbs—Generally, any part of a plant which can be used as a medical treatment, nutrient, food seasoning, or dye. However, this definition is too shortsighted to be relevant to the needs of otherwise healthy athletes whose major objective in life is to excel in their respective sports.

high-density lipoprotein (HDL)—A type of lipoprotein that seems to provide protection against the buildup of atherosclerotic fat deposits in the arteries, HDL contains high levels of protein and low levels of triglycerides and cholesterol. Exercise seems to increase the HDL fraction of total cholesterol.

hop (*Humulus lupulus*)—Plant that can be used as a mild sedative, muscle relaxer, hypnotic, and astringent. Hops also have anti-microbial properties.

horsetail grass (*Equisetum arvense*)—Herb containing alkaloids and flavonoids, which make it an excellent diuretic and astringent for the urinary system.

hydrangea (*Hydrangea arborescens*)—Plant used in the treatment of inflamed prostate glands. It also can be used in the treatment of urinary stones.

hydroxycitrate (HCA)—A natural fruit acid found in abundance in the brindall berry, the fruit of the garcinia cambogia plant found primarily in India. HCA, sometimes referred to as hydroxycitric acid, is cited in research as able to inhibit fat synthesis. Possible mechanisms for this effect may be an appetite-suppressant response due to enhanced gluconeogenesis which would promote a feeling of satiety, and inhibition of certain enzymes necessary for biosynthesizing fat.

hypnotics—Agents that gently and quickly induce sleep and improve the quality of sleep, which also can affect growth hormone output and recovery from workouts and injuries.

hypotensives—Agents that help normalize blood pressure.

hyssop (*Hyssopus officinalis*)—Plant containing terpenoids, flavonoids, tannins, and volatile oils. Hyssop can be used as an anti-spasmodic, expectorant, diaphoretic, nervine, anti-inflammatory, carminative, and hepatic. Its most common use is as a remedy for coughs and bronchitis.

inosine—A naturally occurring compound found in the body that contributes to strong heart-muscle contraction and blood flow in the coronary arteries. As a supplement taken before and during workouts and competition, it stimulates enzyme activity in both cardiac and skeletal muscle cells for improved regeneration of ATP.

inositol—A B-complex vitamin. It combines with choline to form lecithin, protecting against the fatty hardening of arteries and cholesterol buildup. Inositol is important in the nutrition of brain cells and promotes healthy hair. No RDA. Dietary sources include liver, brewer's yeast, dried lima beans, beef brains and heart, and cantaloupe.

insulinlike growth factors (IGF-I and IGF-II)—Substances theorized to be liberated into the interstitial spaces surrounding muscle cells, especially Type IIb fibers, damaged by severe stress such as eccentric contractions. Their collective function is to ensure fusion between the nearby satellite cells with the damaged fiber, thereby decreasing that fiber's proneness to injury. It is theorized to be the single most contributory factor in muscle hypertrophy.

insulinomimetics—Herbs used for their apparent ability to simulate the action of insulin. Among these, pterocarpus marsupium, long used by Ayurvedic practitioners in India for treating diabetes, is believed to be capable of regenerating damaged cells in the pancreas where insulin is synthesized. Momordica charantia, fenugreek, and bilberry contain insulinlike polypeptides shown to help reduce high blood sugar. And specially prepared extracts from onion and garlic plants have been clinically shown to reduce blood glucose by competing with insulin for insulin-inactivating compounds, thereby increasing free insulin in body. These powerful botanicals are reported to lower blood pressure, reduce cholesterol, and provide general cardiovascular benefits.

iodine—An essential element for the function of the thyroid gland, which regulates metabolism and energy. Dietary sources include all seafood and kelp. Some brands of table salt have also been supplemented with iodine.

iron—Substance that combines with protein and copper to make hemoglobin, a pigment that colors the blood red and carries oxygen through the bloodstream from the lungs to all bodily tissue. Iron also forms myoglobin, which transports oxygen in muscle tissue for use in fueling contractions. Iron is easily lost through sweat, urine, feces, and menstrual flow. Runners in particular are suspected of inefficiently absorbing dietary iron. Dietary sources includes liver, oysters, lean meat, leafy green vegetables, whole grains, dried fruits, and legumes.

juniper berry (*Juniperus communis*)—Herb used as an antiseptic in a variety of conditions involving the kidney. It can also improve overall kidney functioning.

kava kava (*Piper methysticum*)—Herb named by South Seas islanders who make a drink of it to take in their religious ceremonies. The drink causes calmness and relaxation, with enhanced mental activity. Kava kava appears to be without narcotic action. The active constituents in the root are lactones called kava pyrones, which, in high doses, depress the central nervous system at the level of the reticular formation of the brain stem, and relax the skeletal muscles.

KIC—*See* **alpha ketoisocaproate**.

kola nut (*Cola vera*)—Plant containing caffeine and tannins. It can be used to stimulate the central nervous system and as an antidepressive. *See* **caffeine**.

L-carnitine—Neither an amino acid nor a vitamin but a derivative of hydroxybutyric acid. It is naturally obtained from red meat, and helps release stored body fat into the bloodstream for use in cellular energy processing. Its physiological role is to transport long-chain fatty acids into the mitochondria for energy production. This is believed to improve one's fat metabolism and long-term energy level. Research has also shown L-carnitine to have a value in treating certain cardiovascular disorders, including hardening of the arteries.

lactose—A disaccharide of milk, which on hydrolysis yields glucose and galactose. Bacteria can convert it into lactic acid and butyric acid, as in the souring of milk. It is used in infant feeding formulas, in other foods, and as an osmotic laxative and diuretic. Lactose is not tolerated in many persons after weaning, owing to a reduced lactase activity.

lavender (*Lavandula officinalis*)—Herb often used for culinary or cosmetic purposes and effective for treating headaches and relieving many symptoms of stress. It can also be used as a mild tonic for the nervous system.

laxatives—Agents that stimulate bowel movement to remove wastes and toxins from the body. Laxatives are a multimillion-dollar business for the pharmaceutical industry. Many herbs also serve as laxatives and are much gentler on the body than commercial brands. They're also a lot less expensive. With all laxatives, however, bodily fluids and vital minerals are also lost. So, as with diuretics, use caution when taking laxative herbs. Do not prolong laxative use.

lemon (*Citrus limon*)—Fruit that can be used to treat a number of ailments, including colds, sore throats, and coughs. When the juice is externally applied, it can help soothe sunburns.

lemon balm (*Melissa officinalis*)—Plant that removes spasms and tension which might prevent sleep. It also can provide a morning energy boost. Lemon balm is a good neural sedative and is combined with valerian, hops, and passionflower in a German proprietary medicine that improve the ability to fall asleep.

lemongrass (*Cymbopogon citratus*)—Plant commonly used in soaps and baths to treat oily skin.

licorice root (*Glycyrrhiza glabra*)—Plant that is useful in preventing stomach ulcers, reducing cholesterol levels, and as a stimulant for the liver and the circulatory system. It is also used for its anti-inflammatory and anti-arthritic properties, and has a beneficial effect on the gastrointestinal tract by inhibiting gastric acid secretion.

linden flowers (*Tilia europea*)—Herb containing volatile oils and flavonoids which can help relieve nervous tension. As a result, linden can be used in the treatment of arteriosclerosis and hypertension.

linoleic acid—An essential unsaturated fatty acid which brings oxygen to all cells, tissues, and organs through the blood. It maintains the resilience and lubrication of all cells, and combines with protein and cholesterol to form living membranes which hold body cells together. It also helps regulate the rate of blood coagulation and breaks up cholesterol deposited on arterial walls. Linoleic acid cannot be synthesized in many species and therefore must be provided in the diet. Corn, safflower, and soybean oils are high in linoleic acid, which should provide about 2 percent of total dietary calories.

linolenic acid—An essential fatty acid found in vegetables, peanut oil, and other plants. A linolenic acid deficiency will result in hair loss, poor wound healing, and scaly dermatitis. Linolenic acid is used in the manufacture of paints, coatings, and vitamins, and used therapeutically as some vitamins.

lipoprotein—Combination of a lipid and protein. Cholesterol is transported in the blood plasma by lipoproteins.

low-density lipoprotein (LDL)—A lipoprotein carrying a high level of cholesterol, moderate levels of protein, and low levels of triglycerides. Associated with the building of atherosclerotic deposits in the arteries.

ma huang (*Ephedra sinica*)—Herb shown to be useful as a vasodilatory, hypertensive, circulatory stimulant, anti-allergic, powerful bronchodilator, and in reducing joint pain. It is the source of ephedrine, one of the main medicines for asthma attacks. It is extremely useful for its nasal decongestant properties as well.

magnesium—A pivotal mineral important to protein synthesis, energy production, muscle contractions, and a strong heart muscle. Magnesium is essential for metabolism of calcium, phosphorus, sodium, potassium, and vitamin C. Chronic muscle cramps are a typical sign of magnesium deficiency. Dietary sources include figs, lemons, grapefruit, yellow corn, almonds, nuts, seeds, and dark green vegetables.

manganese—A key enzyme activator. Manganese is also vital to the formation of thyroid and reproductive hormones, normal skeletal development, muscle reflexes, and the proper digestion and utilization of food. Dietary sources include whole grains, egg yolks, nuts, seeds, and green vegetables.

maria thistle—Herb containing the active compound silymarin. It is known to protect and restore normal metabolic function to the liver, promote cellular regeneration via increased protein synthesis, and aid in protecting the kidneys. It also acts as a powerful antioxidant, principally through its sparing effects on glutathione, which also probably accounts for its potency in improving liver function.

milk thistle (*Carduus marianum*)—Herb used as a liver and gall bladder tonic. It can be used in protecting the liver from harmful chemicals such as alcohol.

minerals—Substances ingested through food and water, which combine with other basic food components to form enzymes. Minerals, like vitamins, are necessary for life, but there are 96 times more minerals in the body than vitamins. Many minerals are deficient in the diet because of mineral-poor agricultural soil, the result of intensive farming and long-term use of chemical fertilizers and pesticides.

monounsaturated fat—Dietary fat whose molecules have one double bond open to receive more hydrogen. It is found in many nuts, olive oil, and avocados.

motherwort (*Leonurus cardiaca*)—Herb often compared to valerian root for its hypotensive and sedative properties. Recent studies have concluded that motherwort is as much as three times as powerful as valerian root as a hypotensive and cardiac tonic. The active ingredient in motherwort seems to be an alkaloid called leonurin. Because it has sedative and hypotensive properties, it may be wise to avoid motherwort when using drugs which act on the central nervous system.

nervines—Substances that have beneficial effects on the nervous system—the brain, central nervous system, and neuromuscular system, as well as the sympathetic and parasympathetic nervous systems, which bring impulses to and from your body's organs and systems.

nicotine—An alkaloid found in the tobacco plant. Nicotine first stimulates the central nervous system, then depresses it. It is absorbed easily through the mucous membranes and the skin, and is highly toxic. Toxicity symptoms include nausea, vomiting, twitching, and convulsions. Nicotine is used as an agricultural insecticide.

nordihydroguaiaritic acid (NDGA)—The primary active constituent of the chaparral bush, which grows in the southwestern United States and may live more than 1,000 years, NDGA is widely known in the scientific community as a powerful antioxidant, and has the official designation as a "lipoxygenase inhibitor." Both research and folklore classify NDGA as effective in cellular respiration, analgesic activity, anti-inflammatory activity, and vasodepressant activity. These functions make NDGA a potent anti-aging substance.

nutriceutical—A cross between the words *nutritional* and *pharmaceutical*. A nutriceutical is any nutritional supplement designed for any specific clinical purpose. Thus, engineered foods such as Ensure, Enfamil, Nutriment, Met-Rx, and IGF-33 are regarded as nutriceuticals. Due to FDA and FTC regulations, clinical or medical claims cannot be made for them. Thus, all are sold as foods for general consumption or health foods to be used as diet supplements. Medical doctors frequently utilize these and other nutritional supplements in clinical settings.

nutrients—Food and its specific elements and compounds that can be used by the body to build and maintain itself and to produce energy. Conventionally, nutrients refers to the macronutrients (water, protein, fats, carbohydrates) and the micronutrients (vitamins, minerals, trace elements) that are essential for energy and growth. Legally, the term specifically excludes substances that cure or prevent disease, or other clinical functions beyond growth and energy.

oat fiber (*Avena sativa*)—Plant that may be useful in reducing cholesterol, preventing heart disease, and calming an upset stomach.

octacosanol—The active, energy-boosting component of wheat germ oil, which is known to improve endurance, reaction time, and storage of muscle glycogen.

onion (*Allium cepa*)—Plant with an international reputation as a remedy for lowering blood pressure and generally improving the health of the cardiovascular system. Onions also possess the ability to reduce the tendency for unnecessary clotting to occur within the blood vessels. Traditional use of onions in the treatment of hypertension is being supported by research.

ornithine—Substance produced in the urea cycle by splitting off the urea from arginine and converting into citrulline. On decomposition it gives rise to putrescine. It has been demonstrated to be of value as a growth hormone stimulator when administered intravenously; there is no solid evidence that it stimulates growth hormone to a significant degree—enough to stimulate muscle growth—when taken orally.

ornithine alphaketoglutarate (OKG)—Substance clinically shown to decrease muscle protein catabolism, improve nitrogen retention in muscle tissue, augment muscle tissue polyamine response, mediate insulin increase, improve protein synthesis and wound healing in muscles, and promote muscle-building processes. Clinically, OKG is successfully used in treating burn patients as well as traumatized, surgical, and malnourished individuals. There's no doubt about its tissue-building properties in clinical use. While no studies have been reported on its use as a supplement for athletes, it's logical to infer that OKG will aid in building muscle mass and greatly improve post-workout adaptation and recovery processes.

parsley (*Petroselinum sativum*)—Plant rich in many vitamins and minerals, particularly vitamin A, of which it packs almost eight-fold the amount in carrots. Vitamin A is particularly important to athletes. It is used by the liver in the assembly of newly digested amino acids into protein molecules for delivery throughout the body. A vitamin deficiency can result in a lessened ability to build and repair muscle tissue.

passiflora coerulea—Plant containing a phytochemical called chrysin, which has been clinically shown to increase luteinizing hormone (LH). *See* **balm**.

passionflower (*Passiflora incarnata*)—Herb with a widespread reputation for treating sleeplessness, chronic insomnia, stress, and anxiety.

peppermint (*Mentha piperita*)—Plant used as an aid for digestion, gas, and bile flow and in healing the stomach and liver. The active constituents are found in its essential oil, mainly menthol and carvone. The oil's digestion-enhancing properties have been experimentally verified. Experiments conducted in Russia showed improved bile output and gallbladder contraction, both of which stimulate improved digestion. As an aromatic tea, it has a reputation for calming, cleansing, and strengthening the entire body.

peridoxine alphaketoglutarate (**PAK**)—Vitamin B-6, which is ironically combined with the complexing agent alphaketoglutarate to form a high-energy compound. It is widely used as a nutritional supplement to improve energy output.

phosphorus—Substance that works with calcium to build bones and teeth. Provides a key element in the production of ATP. Dietary sources include animal protein and whole grains.

polyunsaturated fat—Dietary fat whose molecules have more than one double bond open to receive more hydrogen. It is found in safflower oil, corn oil, soybeans, sesame seeds, and sunflower seeds.

potassium—Substance that teams with sodium to regulate the body's water balance and heart rhythms. Nerve and muscle function are disturbed when the two minerals are not balanced. Insufficient potassium can lead to fatigue, cramping, and muscle damage. Physical and mental stress, excessive sweating, alcohol, coffee, and a high intake of salt and sugar deplete potassium. Dietary sources include citrus, cantaloupe, green leafy vegetables, and bananas.

potato (*Solanum tuberosum*)—Plant that may help speed healing process of bruises. Potatoes are rich in potassium chloride, which is highly effective in healing bruises.

protein—One of the three basic foodstuffs, along with carbohydrates and fat. Protein is a complex substance present in all living organisms. It comprises 90 percent of the dry weight of blood, 80 percent of muscles, and 70 percent of the skin. Protein provides the connective and structural building blocks of tissue and primary constituents of enzymes, hormones, and antibodies. The components of protein are amino acids. Dietary protein is derived from both animal and plant foods. Protein is essential for growth, the building of new tissue, and the repair of injured or broken-down tissue. It serves as enzymes, structural elements, hormones, immunoglobulins, etc., and is involved in oxygen transport and other activities throughout the body, and in photosynthesis. Protein can be oxidized in the body, liberating heat and energy at the rate of four calories per gram.

psyllium husk (*Plantago ovati*)—Plant that, combined with other herbs, can help ease gastrointestinal disorders and constipation.

pyruvic acid—The end product of the glycolytic pathway. This three-carbon metabolite is an important junction point for two reasons: it is the gateway to the final common energy-producing pathway, the Krebs cycle; and it provides acetyle coenzyme A, through which fatty acids, and in turn fat, are produced from glucose. Pyruvic acid converts to lactic acid as needed. Because thiamine is essential for its oxidation, pyruvic acid increases in the blood and tissues with thiamine deficiency.

red clover (*Trifolium pratense*)—Plant used as a remedy for skin disorders. As an expectorant and antispasmodic, it can also be a useful treatment for coughs and bronchitis.

rhubarb (*Rheum officinale*)—Plant used as a mild lower gastrointestinal tract stimulant, as an appetite stimulant, and to aid in preventing anemia. It has been used in combination with other herbs as a mild laxative. Along with its use as a laxative, rhubarb has been used to stop digestive tract bleeding for more than 1,700 years, and it also has antibiotic properties.

rosemary (*Rosmarinus officinalis*)—Herb containing aromatic volatile oils which reduce inflammation in the intestinal walls. By doing this, rosemary promotes proper functioning of the digestive system, relieves intestinal pain, and removes gas. As a calmative, the effects on the digestive system will promote better nutrients absorption as well as help relieve upset stomach.

royal jelly—Substance produced in the pharyngeal glands of some bees. It is highly nutritional, containing all the B-complex vitamins as well as vitamins A,C, D, and E. Royal jelly is known to relieve several disorders including asthma, liver disease, pancreatitis, insomnia, and stomach and kidney disorders, and it helps the immune system. It must be combined with honey and refrigerated to preserve its potency.

rubefacients—Agents that stimulate blood flow near the skin when applied topically. Because of this action, rubefacients are useful for most athletes because they promote healing and reduce the symptoms of arthritis, joint, and muscle pain.

sage (*Salivia officinalis*)—Herb historically used as a cure-all. Sage is good for digestive disorders, stomach cramps, and gas. Combined with rosemary and peppermint, it can have a calming effect on the body.

sarsaparilla (*Smilax officinalis*)—Herb found to have a general tonic effect that, like Siberian ginseng, has adaptogenic qualities.

saturated fat—Dietary fat from primarily animal sources. Excessive consumption is the major dietary contributor to total blood cholesterol levels and is linked to increased risk for coronary heart disease.

saturated fatty acid—An acid which, by definition, has no available bonds in its hydrocarbon chain; all bonds are filled or saturated with hydrogen atoms. Thus the chain of a saturated fatty acid contains no double bond. Saturated fatty acids are more slowly metabolized by the body than are the unsaturated fatty acids. They include acetic acid, myristic acid, palmitic acid, and steric acid. These acids come primarily from animal sources, with the exception of coconut oil, and are usually solid at room temperature. (Vegetable shortening and margarine have undergone a process called hydrogenation, in which the unsaturated oils are converted to a more solid form.) Other principal sources of saturated fats are milk products and eggs.

saw palmetto (*Serenoa serrulata*)—Plant used as a diuretic, urinary antiseptic, and endocrine agent. It can help strengthen the male reproductive system and may increase low male sex hormones.

selenium—A major nutrient antioxidant along with vitamins A, C, and E. Dietary sources include wheat germ, bran, and tuna.

Siberian ginseng (*Eleutherococcus senticosus*)—A cousin of oriental traditional ginseng, Siberian ginseng has been clinically shown to increase stamina and endurance, speed recovery from workouts, and improve reflexes and concentration, particularly in longer endurance events. It has also been used to treat anemia, depression, and cardiovascular conditions.

simple carbohydrates—Monosaccharides and disaccharides occurring naturally in fruits, vegetables, and dairy products. Some examples of simple carbohydrates are glucose, galactose, and fructose, all of which are monosaccharides, and sucrose, lactose, and maltose, all of which are disaccharides. Most simple carbohydrates elevate blood sugar levels rapidly, providing instant energy that is quickly utilized and dissipated. Fructose is an exception. Additionally, refined sources of simple carbohydrates, such as candy, contribute only calories to the diet. These empty calories are often consumed in place of foods which would provide important nutrients in addition to energy.

skullcap (*Scutellaria laterifolia*)—Herb used in the treatment of nervous tension and in the strengthening of the nervous system. It has also been used in treating seizures and epilepsy.

sodium—An essential mineral for proper growth, and nerve and muscle tissue function. A diet high in salt (40 percent of salt is sodium) causes a potassium imbalance and is associated with high blood pressure. Dietary sources include salt, shellfish, celery, beets, and artichokes.

somalata (*Ephedra equisetina*)—The Indian form of ma huang. *See* **ma huang**.

spirulina—An edible, bluish-green algae that occurs in twisted and coiled filaments. Its nutrient density is legendary. It has been used as a food by the ancient Aztecs and in parts of North Africa.

St. John's wort (*Hypericum perforatum*)—Herb that can be taken as a mild sedative as well as a pain reliever. It has also been used in the treatment of anxiety, tension, varicose veins, and depression, and for wound healing.

starch—A polysaccharide made of glucose linked together. The body must convert starch into glucose, which can be utilized for immediate energy or converted to glycogen and stored in the liver for later energy needs. It exists throughout the vegetable kingdom, but its chief commercial sources are cereals and potatoes.

succinates—Acids with varied biological activities. Their chief function is in their enzyme activity, but they also combine with protein to rebuild muscle fiber and nerve endings, and to help fight infection.

sucrose—A sweet disaccharide that occurs naturally in most land plants and is the simple carbohydrate obtained from sugarcane, sugar beet, and other sources. It is hydrolyzed in the intestine by sucrase to glucose and fructose.

sulfur—A mineral of major structural importance to proteins, enzymes, antibodies, skin, and hair. Dietary sources include beans, beef, and eggs.

supplements—Any enterally (taken into the body by mouth) or parenterally (taken into the body other than by mouth) administered substance which serves health, growth, or other bodily processes that food alone either cannot accomplish or cannot accomplish as efficiently. Supplements can be nutritional or non-nutritional in nature. The traditionally identified classifications of supplements are health foods, additives, herbals, nutriceuticals, micronutrients, macronutrients, adaptogens, ergogenic compounds, and anabolic compounds.

tea tree oil (*Melaleuca alternifolia*)—Plant containing some antiseptic properties. It has been shown to be effective on a variety of skin sores, including athlete's foot, burns, canker sores, cuts, bruises, and abrasions when applied to the sore. It has also been used as a skin disinfectant and causes no reported irritation to the skin.

tieh ta yao gin—A mild liniment for sprains, strains, deep bone bruises, and hairline fractures. It has been used as an anesthesia for reducing dislocations.

tiger balm—Oil containing menthol, wintergreen, eucalyptus, and lavender oil, among other ingredients. It has been known to soothe minor aches and pains, toothaches, and itching.

tonics—Agents that vitalize and nourish either one organ of the body or the entire body. Unlike chemical drugs, tonics help prevent health problems and can be taken with very little worry of side effects or overdose. While tonics should be used in times of good health, they can be especially helpful if signs of illness start to appear.

tribulus (*Tribulus terrestris*)—*See* **goathead**.

triglyceride—A combination of glycerol with three fatty acids: stearic acid, oleic acid, and palmitic acid.

tumeric (*Curcuma longa*)—Herb containing the phytochemical curicumin. Curicumin has been shown to be a more powerful anti-inflammatory than ibuprofen and as effective as cortisone.

ubiquinone—*See* **coenzyme Q-10**.

unsaturated fatty acids (UFA)—Acids that are important in lowering blood cholesterol and may thus help prevent heart disease. They are essential for normal glandular activity, healthy skin and mucous membranes, and many metabolic processes. UFA are fatty acids whose carbon chain contains one or more double or triple bonds, and which are capable of receiving more hydrogen atoms. They include the group polyunsaturates, are generally liquid at room temperature, and are derived from vegetables, nuts, seeds, or other sources. Examples of unsaturated fatty acids include corn oil, safflower oil, sunflower oil, and olive oil. Replacing saturated fats with unsaturated fats in the diet can help reduce cholesterol levels. A small amount of highly unsaturated fatty acid is essential to animal nutrition. The body cannot desaturate a fat, such as vegetable shortening or margarine, sufficiently by its own metabolic processes to supply this essential need. Therefore, the dietary inclusion of unsaturated or polyunsaturated fats is vital. *See* **essential fatty acids**.

uva ursi—A bitter herb which has been used for kidney and bladder infections. It also has properties which strengthen the heart, spleen, liver, and small intestines, has diuretic properties, and is good for female disorders.

valerian root (*Valerian officinalis*)—Herb used historically as a mild, natural sedative, and for its ability to aid in mental concentration and improved coordination. Its calming effect, it seems, also aids digestion.

vanadyl sulfate (voso4)—Sulfate extensively studied for its insulin-like activity as a blood glucose–lowering agent. In other words, vanadyl sulfate increases glucose uptake by muscle cells. Its benefits include increased energy for workouts, more rapid recovery following workouts, increased muscle glycogen that results in better muscle growth and repair, and increased glycogen storage providing a fuller, more dense muscle appearance. Care must be taken with voso4, however. Vanadium can build up in various tissues of the body, especially the kidneys. The chelators capable of reducing this danger are vitamin C, glutathione, and other antioxidants.

vitamins—Organic food substances present in plants and animals that are essential in small quantities for the proper functioning of every organ of the body, and for all energy production. Most are obtained from food, but supplementation is almost always advised and regarded as critical for athletes in heavy training.

vitamin A—A fat-soluble vitamin occurring as preformed vitamin A (retinol), found in animal-origin foods, and provitamin A (carotene), provided by both plant and animal foods. Vitamin A maintains healthy skin, mucous membranes, eyesight, and immune system function, and promotes strong bones and teeth. It is vital to the liver's processing of protein. Dietary sources include fish-liver oil, liver, eggs, milk and dairy products, green and yellow vegetables, and yellow fruits.

vitamin B-1 (*thiamine*)—Vitamin essential for learning capacity and muscle tone in the stomach, intestines, and heart. Dietary sources include brewer's yeast, wheat germ, blackstrap molasses, whole wheat and rice, oatmeal, and most vegetables.

vitamin B-12 (*cobalamin*)—Vitamin necessary for normal metabolism of nerve tissue and formation and regeneration of red blood cells. Dietary source is animal protein, especially liver.

vitamin B-2 (*riboflavin*)—An essential cofactor in the enzymatic breakdown of all foodstuffs. It is important to cell respiration, good vision, skin, and hair. Dietary sources include liver, tongue, organ meats, milk, and eggs. The amount of vitamin B-2 found in foods is minimal, making this America's most common vitamin deficiency.

vitamin B-3 (*niacin*)—Vitamin essential for synthesis of sex hormones, insulin, and other hormones. Effective in improving circulation and reducing blood cholesterol. Dietary sources include lean meats, poultry, fish, and peanuts.

vitamin B-5 (*pantothenic acid*)—An important stress, immune system, and anti-allergy factor. It is vital for proper functioning of adrenal glands, where stress chemicals are produced, and it promotes endurance. Dietary sources include organ meats, egg yolks, and whole-grain cereals.

vitamin B-6 (*pyridoxine*)—Vitamin essential for the production of antibodies and red blood cells, and the proper assimilation of protein. The more protein in the diet, the more B-6 is needed. It facilitates conversion of stored liver and muscle glycogen into energy. Dietary sources include brewer's yeast, wheat bran, wheat germ, liver, kidney, and cantaloupe.

vitamin B complex—The vitamin B complex is comprised of eight related nutrients: thiamin (vitamin B-1), riboflavin (vitamin B-2), niacin (vitamin B-3), pantothenic acid (vitamin B-5), folic acid, biotin, vitamin B-6, and vitamin B-12. Together, the B-complex vitamins are needed for the release of energy from food and for the health of the nervous and digestive systems. They play critical roles in the synthesis and repair of genes and in the maintenance of the skin, hair, and nails. This group of vitamins is not stored in the body and must be replenished on a daily basis. When you exercise strenuously, your body quickly burns up its vitamin B supply. A shortage of B-complex vitamins affects both performance and recovery. High consumption of sugar, caffeine, processed food, and alcohol causes depletion. These vitamins are grouped together because of their common source and distribution, and their interrelationship as coenzymes in metabolic processes. All must be present together for the B-complex to work. The best food source for vitamin B complex is brewer's yeast. Certain other factors associated with the B complex were originally thought to be B vitamins. Choline and inositol are often included in B-complex supplements because they help in fat metabolism in the liver, and they are involved in the formation of acetylcholine, which transmits nerve impulses. Another, para-aminobenzoic acid (PABA) is actually a part of the folic acid molecule. PABA is readily available in food and is made by our intestinal bacteria. It is known specifically for its nourishment to hair and its usefulness as a sunscreen. However, these are not actually true B vitamins.

vitamin C—A critical health-protection nutrient. Body stores of vitamin C are depleted rapidly by drugs, toxins, smoking, exercise, and stress. It fortifies the immune system against virus infections, strengthens blood vessels, reduces cardiovascular abnormalities, and lowers fat and cholesterol levels. As a natural anesthetic vitamin C reduces many kinds of pain. It also helps detoxify chemical and metal contaminants found in the air, water, and food; slows down lactic acid buildup; and helps heal wounds, scar tissue, and injuries. Vitamin C is necessary in the formation of connective tissue. Dietary sources include citrus fruits, berries, green and leafy vegetables, tomatoes, and potatoes.

vitamin D—A fat-soluble vitamin, acquired through sunlight or diet. Vitamin D aids the body in utilization of vitamin A, calcium, and phosphorus. It helps maintain a stable nervous system and normal heart action. Dietary sources include fish-liver oils, sardines, salmon, tuna, and milk and dairy products.

vitamin E—Fat-soluble vitamin and active antioxidant that retards free-radical damage as well as protecting oxidation of fat compounds, vitamin A, and other nutritional factors in the body. It is important to cellular respiration, proper circulation, protecting of lungs against air pollution, and preventing of blood clots. It also helps alleviate leg cramps and charley horses. Dietary sources include wheat germ, cold-pressed vegetable oils, whole raw seeds and nuts, and soybeans.

vitamin K—Vitamin implicated in proper blood clotting. It is synthesized in the intestinal flora. Because it is fat soluble, it has the potential for toxicity if taken in large doses.

vitamin P—*See* **bioflavonoids**.

vulneraries—Category of herbs that promote healing of cuts, abrasions, and bruises; relieve tissue irritations; and promote blood flow to areas affected by bruises and inflamed tissues.

whey—A milk by-product with a biological value of 80–88. In recent years, clinical scientists have improved the biological value by enzymatically altering the bonds between the amino acids forming the whey protein complex. Another method of engineering whey utilizes various filtration techniques.

white willow bark (*Salix alba*)—Herb administered for a number of ailments, including headaches, fever, rheumatism, neuralgia, arthritis, gout, angina, and sore muscles. The pain-relieving substance in white willow bark was first isolated during the 1820s when salicin was isolated and identified. Later, acetylsalicylic acid was produced from salicylic acid and aspirin was born.

wild yam root (*Dioscorea villosa*)—Plant with antispasmodic, anti-inflammatory, antirheumatic, and hepatic properties. It is valuable in the relief of intestinal colic, diverticulitus, and ovarian and uterine pain. It is especially useful in the treatment of rheumatoid arthritis.

wintergreen (*Gaultheria procumben*)—Plant whose oil has long been used to ease headaches, muscle and joint aches, and pain, inflammation, and rheumatism.

wood betony (*Betonica officinalis*)—Herb whose alkaloids and tannins can help strengthen the nervous system and have a relaxing effect. It can also ease anxiety, tension, and headaches.

xiaopangmei (**xpm**)—A Traditional Chinese Medicine (tcm) recently put to a single blind test in which researchers noted a highly significant body-fat reduction in comparison to a control group and a placebo group. Upon further testing researchers discovered this reduction had resulted from inhibiting the brain's appetite center and intestinal absorption of glucose, and strengthened physical capacity. Xpm subjects could swim longer and showed no decrease in muscular strength despite significant weight loss. No side effects were found.

yarrow (*Achillea millefolium*)—Substance with a high concentration of unsaturated fatty acids. It aids the heart by lowering blood cholesterol and may prevent heart disease.

yeast—A one-celled fungus used in brewing and leavening bread. Some yeast, such as brewer's yeast, is highly nutritious, but many individuals are allergic to yeast. Candida albicans is a common yeast living within the body which can multiply and produce sickness-causing toxins. Antibiotics, sugar-rich diets, birth control pills, cortisone, and other drugs stimulate candida growth.

yerba maté (*Ilex paraquariensis*)—South American plant used widely throughout the world to increase mental clarity. Yerba maté contains a huge amount of mateine, a relative to caffeine, but produces none of the latter's undesirable side effects. Also packed with sizable portions of vitamins B-1, B-2, and C, yerba maté has antistress properties and aids nervous-tissue function.

yucca (*Yucca lilianceae*)—Herb whose saponins have long been used by North American Indians to reduce swelling and pain. It is also known to treat gout, urethritis, and prostatitis and as a blood purifier.

zheng gu shui—A powerful liniment for sprains, strains, deep bone bruises, and hairline fractures. It has been used as an anesthesia for treating dislocations.

zinc—Substance that plays a significant role in protein synthesis, maintenance of enzyme systems, contractibility of muscles, formation of insulin, synthesis of DNA, healing processes, prostrate health, and male reproductive fluid. Deficiencies are common due to food processing and zinc-poor soil. Excessive sweating can drain up to three milligrams daily. Dietary sources include meat, wheat germ, brewer's yeast, pumpkin seeds, and eggs. Zinc chelate is the element zinc in supplemental form and coated with protein, thus increasing the likelihood that it can be assimilated by the body.

Zinc deficiency is associated with anemia, short stature, hypogonadism, impaired wound healing, and geophagia. Zinc salts are often poisonous when absorbed by the system, producing a chronic poisoning resembling that caused by lead.

Summary of Important Herbal Tonic Recommendations in This Book

Note: Most of the individual herbs mentioned in this book are available in health food stores specializing in herbs. If you have any problems finding them, or if you are interested in the herbal tonics covered in this book, the authors recommend you contact:

BioBotanica, Inc.
75 Commerce Drive
Hauppauge, NY 11788
(800) 645-5720, (516) 231-5522

Country Life, Inc.
101 Corporate Drive
Hauppauge, NY 11788
(800) 645-5768, (516) 231-1031

Weider Health & Fitness
21100 Erwin Street
Woodland Hills, CA 91365
(818) 884-6800

PB Distributors
65 Dorsett Street
Springfield, MA 01108
PTCHOICE@worldnet.att.net
(800) 732-2004, (413) 734-5642

Developing a Foundation

Most health food stores carry several herbal cleansing formulas. Look at all of them and choose the one that incorporates at least several of the herbs listed. It is not difficult to mix and match several different products, since they are almost always provided in standardized dosages. Remember that each tablet will usually contain equal parts of each herb.

The following blends of cleansing herbs can be used prior to initiating an intense fitness, bodybuilding, or sports-training program:

Blood and Liver

red clover
burdock
rhubarb
goldenseal
milk thistle
licorice
dandelion

Kidney

cornsilk
couch grass
hydrangea
uva ursi
althea root

Colon

psyllium seed
flax seed

Directions: Take three (3) tablets from each of the three cleansing categories in the table above three times daily with meals, for the three days prior to commencing your pre-competition training cycle.

Adaptation Processes

Siberian ginseng
Oriental ginseng
echinacea
goldenseal
mumie
pantocrine
   (reindeer antler)

Muscle Mass

sarsaparilla root
wild yam root
saw palmetto fruit
Siberian ginseng
damiana leaf
avena sativa
licorice root
fenugreek seed

Directions: Take 1–2 ml of the extract three times daily with meals.

Strength and Power

ginkgo biloba	wood betony
yerba maté	avena sativa
blue vervian	

Directions: Take 1–2 ml of the extract three times daily with meals.

Restorative Processes

horsetail grass	fleece flower root
saw palmetto fruit	ginkgo biloba
fenugreek seed	capsicum fruit
teasel root	

Directions: Take 1–2 ml of the extract three times daily with meals.

Antioxidant Formula

green tea extract	maria thistle
Siberian ginseng	gotu kola
ginkgo biloba	capsicum
bilberry	kola nut

Directions: Take 1–2 ml of the extract three times daily with meals.

Fat Loss

brindall berry	evening primrose oil
gymnema sylvestre	acidophilus

Directions: Take 1–2 ml of the extract three times daily with meals.

Heart

hawthorn	motherwort
garlic	ginkgo biloba
linden flowers	night-blooming cereus

yarrow   una de gato
borage   onion

Directions: Take 1–2 ml of the extract three times daily with meals.

Digestion and Assimilation

ginger   cardamom
gentian root   valerian root
bitter orange   licorice
dandelion   cayenne
angelica   peppermint
rhubarb

Directions: Take 1–2 ml of the extract three times daily with meals.

Prestart Phenomenon

kava kava   black cohosh
valerian root   skullcap
passionflower   hops
wood betony   ginger root

Directions: Take 2–4 ml of the extract 30 minutes before competing.

Nervous System

oats   valerian
skullcap   ashwagandha
St. John's wort   chamomile
motherwort   gotu kola
lobelia   fo-ti

Directions: Take 2–4 ml of the extract before your skill workout.

Better Sleep

valerian root	passionflower
skullcap	royal jelly
hops	

Directions: Take 2–4 ml of the extract 20 minutes before bedtime.

Sports Injuries

gotu kola	St. John's wort
fo-ti	marigold
comfrey	ginger
chamomile	aloe vera

Directions: Take 1–2 ml of the extract just before each meal.

Pain

white willow bark	ashwagandha
yucca	

Directions: Take 2–4 ml of the extract as needed for pain. Do NOT exceed four times daily.

Mental Focus

ginkgo biloba	wood betony
yerba maté	oat
blue vervian	

Directions: Take 2–4 ml of the extract before competition or practice.

Energy

inulin	licorice

yerba maté   codonopsis
blueberry leaf   astragalus

Directions: Take 2–4 ml of the extract before competition or practice. (Caution: Do *not* engage in the use of herbs such as ma huang and similar stimulants, as they are powerful and banned by most sports federations.)

Preventive Health

cardiovascular—hawthorn, garlic, ginkgo
respiratory—mullein, elecampane
digestive and intestinal tracts—bitters, una de gato
liver—bitters, milk thistle
urinary—buchu, uva ursi
women's reproductive—raspberry
men's reproductive—saw palmetto or damiana
nervous system—oats, skullcap, St. John's wort
musculoskeletal—celery seed, nettle
skin—cleavers, nettle, red clover
immune system—una de gato, echinacea, goldenseal

Directions: Use the recommended herbs as symptoms dictate. It is always best to consult with a qualified herbalist before embarking on an herbal approach to better health or treating medical conditions.

Stimulants for Different Parts of the Body

Circulatory system: stimulating blood flow isn't always a good idea, particularly if you have heart problems. For otherwise healthy athletes, however, it can reap dividends. Bayberry, ginseng, prickly ash, rosemary, rue, wormwood, and yarrow may stimulate circulation.

Respiratory system: the diaphoretics—which stimulate improved breathing—include angelica, balm of gilead, benzoin, eucalyptus, garlic, ground ivy, horseradish, mustard, peppermint, sage, white horehound, and yarrow.

Digestive system: bitters may be considered as stimulants to improve digestive processes. Balmony, bayberry, caraway, cardamom, cinnamon, coffee, dandelion root, galangal, garlic, gentian, horseradish, mustard, peppermint, rosemary, rue, and wormwood are common bitters.

Urinary system: cayenne is the best stimulant for the urinary system, but we can add eucalyptus, gravel root, juniper, and yarrow.

Muscles: ginger and cayenne are excellent stimulants to peripheral circulation. Mustard and horseradish can be included.

Nervous system: nervous system stimulants include cola, guarana, coffee, tea, and yerba maté.

APPENDIX C
Alphabetical Listing of Herb Associations in the United States

Alternative Medical Association
7909 SE Stark Street
Portland, OR 97215
(503) 254-7555

American Alliance of Aromatherapy
PO Box 309
Depoe Bay, OR 93741
(800) 809-9850

American Association of Acupuncture and Oriental Medicine
433 Front Street
Catasaqua, PA 18032-2526
(610) 266-1433;
fax (610) 264-2768

American Association of Naturopathic Physicians
2366 Eastlake Avenue East
Suite 322
Seattle, WA 98102

American Botanical Council
PO Box 144345
Austin, TX 78714-4345
(512) 926-4900;
fax (512) 926-2345;
custserve@herbalgram.org

American Dianthus Society
Rand B. Lee, President
PO Box 22232
Santa Fe, NM 87502-2232
(505) 438-7038; randbear@nets

American Ginseng Society, Inc.
PO Box 754
Brookly, MI 49230-0754

American Herb Association
PO Box 1673
Nevada City, CA 95959
(916) 265-9552

American Herbal Products Association
PO Box 30585
Bethesda, MD 20824
(301) 951-3207

The American Herbalists Guild
PO Box 746555
Arvada, CO 80006
(303) 423-8800;
fax (303) 423-8828;
ahg@earthlink.net

**American Holistic Health
Association**
Suzan Walter, President
PO Box 17400
Anaheim, CA 92817-7400
(714) 779-6152

**American Holistic Medical
Association**
4101 Lake Boone Trail
Suite 201
Raleigh, NC 27607
(919) 787-5146;
fax (919) 787-4916

**American Holistic Nurses'
Association**
4101 Lake Boone Trail
Suite 201
Raleigh, NC 27602
(919) 787-5181

**American Society for
Horticultural Science**
701 North Saint Asaph Street
Alexandria, VA 22314
(703) 836-4606

**American Society of
Pharmacognosy**
PO Box 9558
Downers Grove, IL 60515
(708) 971-6417;
fax (708) 971-6097

**Association for the Promotion
of Herbal Healing**
George Weissman
PO Box 7011
Berkeley, CA 94707
(415) 526-6250

**Association of Natural
Medicine Pharmacists**
8369 Camps de Elysses
Forestville, CA 95436
(707) 887-1351;
fax (707) 887-9094

**Bio-Dynamic Farming and
Gardening Association, Inc.**
PO Box 550
Kimberton, PA 19442
(620) 935-7797

**Dr. Edward Bach Healing
Society**
Karen Maresca
644 Merrick Road
Lynbrook, NY 11563
(516) 593-2206,
(800) 433-7523

Flower Essence Society
Richard Katz
PO Box 459
Nevada City, CA 95959
(800) 736-9222,
(916) 256-9163;
fax (916) 265-0584;
info@flowersociety.org

Fragrance Foundation
Annette Green
145 East 32nd Street
New York, NY 10016

Garlic Seed Foundation
David Stern, Director
Rose Valley Farm
Rose, NY 14542-0149
(315) 587-9787

The Herb and Botanical Alliance
Anita Beckwith
5916 Duerer Street
PO Box 93
Egg Harbor, NJ 08215-0093
(609) 965-0337;
fax (609) 965-4488

Herb Research Foundation
Rob McCaleb
1007 Pearl Street
Suite 200
Boulder, CO 80302
(303) 449-2265;
fax (303) 449-7849

Herb Society of America
David Pauer, Executive Director
Michelle Milks,
Administrative Assistant
9019 Kirtland-Chardon Road
Kirtland, OH 44094
(216) 256-0514;
fax (216) 256-0541

Homeopathic Education Services
2124 Kittredge Street
Berkeley, CA 94704
(510) 649-0294

Hydroponic Society of America
2819 Crow Canyon Road
Suite 218
San Ramon, CA 94583
(510) 743-9605

International Aloe Science Council
415 East Airport Freeway
Suite 365
Irving, TX 75062
(214) 258-8772;
fax (214) 258-8777

International Aromatherapy and Herb Association
Jeffrey Schiller
3541 West Acapulco Lane
Phoenix, AZ 85023
(602) 938-4439;
jeffreys@aztec.asu.edu

International Herb Association
Southeastern Regional Chapter
Dell Ratcliffe, the Country
Shepherd
Rt. 1, Box 107
Comer, GA 30629
(706) 788-3166;
mfzx30a@prodigy.com

**National Association for
Holistic Aromatherapy**
836 Hanely Ind. Court
St. Louis, MO 63144
(888) ASK-NAHA;
fax (314) 963-4454,
(314) 963-2071; info@naha.org

**National Nutritional Foods
Association**
3931 MacArthur Boulevard
Suite 101
Newport Beach, CA 92660
(714) 622-6272;
fax (714) 622-6266

**National Oils Research
Association**
894H Route 52
Beacon, NY 12508
(914) 838-4340
(phone and fax);
norassoc@aol.com

Natural Food Associates
PO Box 210
Atlanta, TX 75551

**New Age Publishing and
Retailing Association (NAPRA)**
PO Box 9
Eastsound, WA 98245
(206) 376-2702

Northeast Herbal Association
Ann Hort, Secretary
PO Box 10
Newport, NY 13416
neha@jeansgreens.com

Society of Ethnobiology
Brien A. Meilleur,
Secretary, treasurer
Center for Plant Conservation
Missouri Botanical Garden
PO Box 299
St. Louis, MO 63166

Western Reserve Herb Society
11030 East Boulevard
Cleveland, OH 44106

The Xerces Society
Melody Mackey Allen
10 Southwest Ash Street
Portland, OR 97204
(503) 222-2788;
fax (503) 222-2763

Bibliography

American Herbalist Guild. *American Herbalism: Essays on Herbs and Herbalism.* Freedom, CA: Crossing Press, 1992.

Anderson, F. J. *An Illustrated History of the Herbals.* New York, NY: Columbia University Press, 1985.

Awoniyi, C., et al. "Regulation of Gonadotropin Secretion in the Male: Effect of an Aromatization Inhibitor in Estradiol-Implanted, Orchidectomized Dogs." *Journal of Andrology* vol. 7 (1986): 243–239.

Balch, J. F., and P. A. Balch. *Prescription for Nutritional Healing.* Garden City Park, NY: Avery Publishing, 1990.

Belch, J. F., and D. Ansell, L. Curan, M. McLaren, A. O'Dowd, C. D. Forbes. *The Effects of Efamol and Efamol Marine on Patients with Rheumatoid Arthritis.* Florence, Italy: 6th International Congress on Prostaglandins, 1986.

Benendonk, B. *The Gold, the Glory . . . and the Decay.* Horton, Norway: Hilton Publishing, 1993.

Bland, J. *Medical Applications of Clinical Nutrition.* New Canaan, CT: Keats, 1983.

———. *Nutraerobics.* San Francisco, CA: Harper & Row, 1983.

Bradlow, H. L., et al. "Indole-3-Carbinol: A Novel Approach to Breast Cancer Prevention." *Annals of New York Academy of Sciences* Vol. 768 (1995): 180–200.

Bradlow, H. L., et al. "Long-Term Responses of Women to Indole-3-Carbinol or a High Fiber Diet," *Cancer Epidemiology Biomarkers Prevention* 3 (1994): 591–595.

Bray, G. A., et al. "Hypothalamic and Genetic Obesity in Experimental Animals: An Autonomic and Endocrine Hypothesis." *Physiology Review* Vol. 59: 719–809.

Bressler, R., M. D. Bogdonoff, and G. J. Subak-Sharpe. *The Physicians Drug Manual.* Garden City, NY: Doubleday & Co., Inc., 1981.

British Bates, D., and P. R. W. Fawcett, D. A. Shaw, D. Weightman. *British Medical Herbal Pharmacopoeia.* Bournemouth, England: British Herbal Medicine Assn., 1990.

Brush, M. G. and R. W. Taylor. *Gammalinolenic Acid (Efamol) in the Treatment of the Premenstrual Syndrome: Clinical Uses of Essential Fatty Acids.* Montreal, Canada: Eden Press, 1982.

Bunce, G. E. "Nutrition and Cataract." *Nutrition Reviews,* 38 (1980).

Carilla, E., et al. "Binding of Permixon, a New Treatment for Prostatic Benign Hyperplasia, to the Cytosolic Androgen Receptor in the Rat Prostate." *Journal of Steroid Biochemistry* vol. 20.1 (1984): 521–523.

Carlotti, P., and D. Gabrielle. *The Cellular Aging Process and Free Radicals.* Sederma, France: DCI, 1989.

Castleman, M. *The Healing Herbs: The Ultimate Guide to the Curative Powers of Homeopathic Pharmacopoeia of the United States* (8th ed., vol. 1). Boston, MA: Otis Committee on Pharmacopoeia of the American Institute of Homeopathy, Clapp and Son, 1981.

Cerutti, P. A. "Prooxidant States and Tumor Promotion." *Science* Vol. 227 (1985): 375–381.

Chasroff, I. J., and J. W. Ellis. *Family Medical Guide.* New York, NY: William Morrow and Company Inc., 1983.

Christensen, P., et al. "Benzodiazepine-Induced Sedation and Cortisol Suppression." *Psychopharmacology* vol. 106 (1992): 511–516.

Cape, Coe, and Rossman. *Fundamentals of Geriatric Medicine.* New York, NY: Raven Press, 1983.

Di Silverio, F., et al. "Evidence That Serenoa Repens Extract Displays Anti-estrogenic Activity in Prostatic Tissue of Benign Prostatic Hypertrophy Patients." *European Eurology* vol. 21.4 (1992): 309–314.

Duke, James A. *CRC Handbook of Medicinal Herbs,* Boca Raton, FL: CRC Press, 1985.

————. *Handbook of Biologically Active Phytochemicals and Their Activities.* Boca Raton, FL: CRC Press, 1992.

————. *Handbook of Edible Weeds.* Boca Raton, FL: CRC Press, 1992.

————. *Handbook of Phytochemical Constituents of Grass, Herbs, and other Economic Plants.* Boca Raton, FL: CRC Press, (1992).

Ellingwood, F. *American Material Medical, Therapeutics & Pharmacognosy.* (1898, repr.) Eclectic Medical Publisher, 1983.

Engasser, P. "Sunscreens," *Journal of American Dermatology.* Jan: 14.

Fishman, J. "Biological Action of Catechol Oestrogens." *Journal of Endocrinology* 89 Supplement (1981): 59P–65P.

Fitzpatrick, F. K. "Plant Substances Active Against Mycobacterium Tuberculosis." *Antibiotics and Chemotherapy* vol. 4, No. 5 (1954): 528–536.

Gastelu, D., and F. C. Hatfield. *Performance Nutrition: The Complete Guide.* Santa Barbara, CA: International Sports Sciences Assn., 1995.

———. *Dynamic Nutrition.* Garden City Park, NY: Avery Publishers.

Glen, E., and I. L. Glen, L. MacDonnell and J. MacKenzie. *Possible Pharmacological Approaches to the Prevention and Treatment of Alcohol Related CNS Impairment: Results of a Double Blind Trial of Essential Fatty Acids.* Inverness: Highland Psychiatric Research Group, Craig Dunain Hospital.

Goodman, L. S., and A. Gilman. *Pharmacy Basis of Therapherapy.* New York, NY: MacMillian, 1975.

Green, J. *The Male Herbal.* Freedom, CA: Crossings Press, 1991.

Grossman, S. P. "Role of the Hypothalmus in the Regulation of Food and Water Intake," *Psychology Review* vol. 82 (1975): 200–224.

Halliwell, B., and J. M. Gutteridge. "Lipid Peroxidation, Oxygen Radicals, Cell Damage, and Antioxidant Therapy." *Lancet,* June 23, 1984.

Hansten, P. D. *Drug Interactions,* 4th ed. Philadelphia, PA: Lea & Febiger, 1979.

Haslett, C., and J. G. Douglas, S. Chalmers, V. E. Weighill, J. F. Munro. *Clinical Uses of Essential Fatty Acids.* Edited by D. F. Horrobin. Montreal, Canada: Eden Press, 1982.

Hatfield, F. C. and E. J. Kreis. *Sports Conditioning: The Complete Guide.* Santa Barbara, CA: International Sports Sciences Assn., 1994.

Hatfield, F. C. and M. Krotee. *Personalized Weight Training for Fitness and Athletics: From Theory to Practice.* Dubuque, IA: Kendall/Hunt Publishers, 1978.

Hatfield, F. C. and M. Yessis. *Oxygen: Its Incredible Story.* Santa Barbara, CA: International Sports Sciences Assn., 1991.

Hatfield, F. C. *Hardcore Bodybuilding: A Scientific Approach.* Chicago, IL: Contemporary Books, 1993.

————. *Fitness: The Complete Guide,* 4th ed. Santa Barbara, CA: International Sports Sciences Assn., 1997.

————. *Power: A Scientific Approach.* Chicago, IL: Contemporary Books, 1989.

————. *Advanced Sports Conditioning.* Tokyo, Japan: Morinaga & Co. 1988.

————. *Ultimate Sports Nutrition.* Chicago, IL: Contemporary Books, 1987.

————. *Ergogenesis: Achieving Peak Athletic Performance Without Drugs.* New Orleans, LA: Fitness Systems, 1985.

————. *Bodybuilding: A Scientific Approach.* Chicago, IL: Contemporary Books, 1983.

————. *Complete Guide to Power Training.* New Orleans, LA: Fitness Systems, 1989.

————. *Powerlifting: A Scientific Approach.* Chicago, IL: Contemporary Books, 1981.

Heinerman, J. *Herbal Dynamics.* Root of Life, Inc., 1982.

Hoffmann, D. *The Elements of Herbalism.* Shaftesbury: Element Books, 1990.

————. *Therapeutic Herbalism.* Sebastopol, CA: Veridtas Press Sebastopol, 1991.

————. *The Herbalist* (multimedia CD-ROM version 2.0M. Hopkins, MN: Hopkins Technology, LLC., 1995.

Holmes, T. H., and R. H. Rahe. "The Social Re-Adjustment Rating Scale." *Journal of Psychomatic Research* Vol. 11 (1967).

Hoorn, R. K. J. and D. Westernik. "Vitamin B-1, B-2 and B-6 Deficiencies in Geriatric Patients." *Clinical Chemistry* 61 (1973).

Hoshino, T., et. al. "Reducing the Photosensitizing Potential of Chlorpromazine with the Simultaneous Use of Beta- and Dimethyl-Beta-Cyclodextrins in Guinea Pigs." *Archives of Dermatological Research* vol. 281, No. 1 (1989): 60–5.

Hudson, J. B. *Antiviral Compounds from Plants.* Boca Raton, FL: CRC Press, 1989.

Ibrahim, A. R. and Y. J. Abul-Hajj. "Aromatase Inhibition by Flavonoids." *Journal of Steroid Biochemistry* vol. 37.2 (1990): 257–260.

Jellinck, P. H., et al. "AH Receptor Binding Properties of Indole Carbinols and Induction of Hepatic Estradiol Hydroxylation." *Biochemistry Pharmacological* Vol. 45.5 (1993): 1129–1136.

Juniewicz, P. E., et al. "Aromatase Inhibition in the Dog. Effect on Serum LH, Serum Testosterone Concentrations, Testicular Secretions and Spermatogenesis," *Journal of Urology* 139.4 (1988): 827–831.

Karimi, Kue, ed. *Nutri-Health Data Computer Program*, Version 4.5. Dallas, TX: Health Data Development, 1990.

Kapoor, K. *CRC Handbook of Ayurvedic Medicinal Plants*. Boca Raton, FL: CRC Press, 1990.

Kastrup, E. K. *Drug Facts and Comparisons*, 1982 ed. Philadelphia, PA; St. Louis, MO: Facts and Comparisons Division, J. P. Lippincott Co., 1982.

Kirsta, A. *The Book of Stress Survival*. Thorsons/HarperCollins, UK.

Kolata, G. "Glaucoma and Cataract: Closing in on Causes." *New York Times*, July 12, 1988.

Kremer, J. M., et al. "Fish Oil Fatty Acid Supplementation in Active Rheumatoid Arthritis." *JAMA* Vol. 258 (1987): 962.

Kronhausen, E., and P. Kronhausen. *Formula for Life*. New York, NY: William Morrow and Co., 1989.

Krotee, M., and F. C. Hatfield. *Theory and Practice of Physical Activity*. Dubuque, IA: Kendall/Hunt Publishers, 1979.

Kunz, J. R. M. *The American Medical Association Family Medical Guide*. New York, NY: Random House, 1982.

Lindeman, R. D. "Mineral Metabolism in the Ageing and Aged." *Journal of American College Nutrition* vol. 1 (1982).

List, P., and L. Hoerhammer. *Hagers Hanbuch der Pharmazeutischen Praxis*, Vols. 2–5. Springer-Verlag, Berlin, 1969.

Lorpela, H., et al. "Effects of Selenium Supplementation After Acute Myocardial Infarction." *Research Communication Chemistry Pathology Pharmacological*. (Finland) vol. 2 (August 1965): 249–52.

Lust, John. *Herb Book*. New York, NY: Bantam Books, 1982.

Mahesh, V. B., and R. B. Greenblatt. "The In Vivo Conversion of Dehydroepiandrosterone and Androstenedione to Testosterone in the Human," *Actual Endocrinology* Vol. 41 (1962): 400–406.

Martens, R. *Coaches Guide to Sports Psychology*. Champaign, IL: Human Kinetics.

McCarron, D. A., and C. D. Morris. "Blood Pressure Response to Oral Calcium in Persons with Mild to Moderate Hypertension. *Annual Internal Medicine* Vol. 103:6, Part 1 (1985): 825–831.

Mabey, R. *The New Age Herbalist.* New York, NY: Macmillan, 1988.

Marsa, L. "Oxygen: New Light on the Free Radicals That Cause Ageing." *Los Angeles Times* (August 28, 1989).

Martin, E. *Drug Interactions Index.* Philadelphia, PA: J. B. Lippincott Co., 1978.

Michnovicz, J. J., and H. L. Bradlow "Altered Estrogen Metabolism and Excretion in Humans Following Consumption of Indole-3-Carbinol." *Nutrition Cancer* vol. 16.1 (1991): 59–66.

Miller and Lindeman. "Red Blood Cell & Serum Selenium Concentration as Influenced by Age & Selected Diseases." *Journal of American College Nutrition* (1983).

Mills, S. *Out of the Earth: The Science and Practice of Herbal Medicine.* New York, NY: Viking Penguin, 1992.

Mills, Simon. *British Herbal Pharmacopoeia.* Bournemouth, England: British Herbal Medicine Assn., 1990.

Mindell, Earl. *Herb Bible.* New York, NY: Simon and Schuster/ Fireside, 1992.

Moore, M. *Medicinal Plants of the Mountain West.* Santa Fe, NM: Museum of New Mexico Press, 1979.

Morrelli, H. F., and K. L. Melmon. "The Clinician's Approach to Drug Interactions." *California Medicine* Vol. 109, No. 1 (1968): 380–389.

Morrison, W. L. "Photoimmunology." *Journal of Investigating Dermatology* Vol. 77 (1981): 73.

Mowrey, D. *Next Generation Herbal Medicine: Guaranteed Potency Herbs.* New Canaan, CT: Keats, 1990.

———. *The Scientific Validation of Herbal Medicine.* New Canaan, CT: Keats, 1990.

———. *Experimental Psychology.* Provo, UT: Brigham Young University, director of Nebo Institute of Herbal Sciences, director of Behavior Change Agent Training Institute, Director of Research, Nova Corp.

Mukhtar, H., et al. "Inhibitory Effects of NDGA on Mutagenicity, Monooxygenase Activities and Cytochrome P-450 and Prostaglandin Synthetase-Dependent Metabolism of Benzo (A)Pyrene (BP)." Meeting abstract, Case Western Reserve University, Cleveland, Federal Proceedings vol. 46, No. 3: 696.

Murray, Michael. *Healing Power of Herbs.* Rocklin, Prima, 1992.

Niwa, Y. "Lipid Peroxides and Superoxide Dimutase (SOD) Induction in Skin Inflammatory Diseases, and Treatment with SOD Preparations." Dermatologica (Japan) vol. 179, Supplement 1 (1989): 101–6.

Pashby, et al. "Clinical Trial of Evening Primrose Oil (Efamol) in Mastalgia. British Surgical Research Society, Cardiff Meeting, July 1981.

Powley, T. L. "The Ventromedial Hypothalmic Syndrome, Satiety and a Cephalic Phase Hypothesis. *Psychology Review* vol. 84 (1977): 89–126.

Qin Zhengyu and Xu Aihua. "Intestinal Absorption of Glucose in Burned Rats and in Alloxin Diabetic Rats," *The Chinese Journal of Burns Plastic Surgery* vol. 4 (1983): 267–269.

——. "Effect of Xiaopangmei (Anti-Obesity Drug) in Rats: A Compilation of Academic Papers and Abstracts of the Beijing International Conference on Sports Medicine." *Chinese Association of Sports Medicine* (1985): 225.

——. "An Experimental Study by Single Blind Method on the Anti-Obesity Effect of Xiaopangmei." *Journal of Traditional Chinese Medicine* vol. 9, no. 1 (1989): 6–8.

Roberts, A. C., et al. "Overtraining Affects Male Reproductive Status." *Fertility Sterility* vol. 60.4 (1993): 686–692.

Robbins, S. L. and R. S. Cotran. *Pathologic Basis of Disease,* 2nd ed. Philadelphia, PA: Saunders Publishing Co., 1979.

Rombi, M. *Phytotherapy: A Practical Handbook of Herbal Medicine.* United Kingdom: Herbal Health Publishers, 1987.

Scientific Committee. *British Herbal Pharmocopaeia.* Lane House, Cowling, Na Keighley, West Yorks: British Herbal Medical Assn., 1983.

Sharma, S. K., and V. P. Singh, R. R. Bhagwat. "In Vitro Antibacterial Effect of the Essential Oil of Oenanthe Javanica (Blume)" *Dc. Indian Journal of Medical Research* vol. 71, No. 1 (1980): 149–151.

Shparer, A. G. and J. W. Marr. "Fatty Acids and Ischaemic Heart Disease." *Lancet* vol. 1 (1978): 1146–1147.

Skalka, H. W., and J. T. Prochal. "Cataracts and Riboflavin Deficiency." *American Journal of Clinical Nutrition* (1981): 34.

Sultan, C., et al. "Inhibition of Androgen Metabolism and Binding by a Liposterolic Extract of 'Serenoa Repens B' in Human Foreskin Fibroblasts." *Journal of Steroid Biochemistry* vol. 20.1 (1984): 515–519.

Taylor, C. R., et. al. "Photoageing/Photodamage and Photoprotection." *American Academy of Dermatology* Vol. 22, No. 1 (Jan. 1990).

Ten Hoor, F. "Cardiovascular Effects of Dietary Linoleic Acid." *Nutrition Metabolism* vol. 24, Supplement 1 (1980): 162–180.

Tierra, L. *The Herbs of Life: Health and Healing Using Western and Chinese Techniques.* Freedom, CA: Crossing Press, 1992.

Tierra, M. *American Herbalism: Essays on Herbs and Herbalism by Members of the American Herbalist Guild.* Freedom, CA: Crossing Press, 1992.

Vaddadi, K. S., and D. F. Horrobin. "Weight Loss Produced by Evening Primrose Oil Administration in Normal and Schizophrenic Individuals." IRCS *Journal of Medicine* vol. 7 (1979): 52.

Wang, S.Y. and C. Merrill, E. Bell. "Effects of Ageing and Long-Term Subcultivation on Collagen Lattice Contraction and Intra-Lattice Proliferation in Three Rat Cell Types." *Mechanical Ageing Development* (Mass. Institute of Technology) vol. 44, no. 2: 127–41.

Werbach, M. R., and M. T. Murray. *Botanical Influences on Illness.* Tarzana, CA: Third Line Press, 1994.

Wills, E. D. "Effects of Antioxidants on Lipid Peroxide Formation in Irradiated Synthetic Diets." *Internal Journal of Radiation Biology* vol. 37, No. 4 (April 1980).

Wolfman, C., et al. "Possible Anxiolytic Effects of Chrysin, a Central Benzodiazepine Receptor Ligand Isolated from Passiflora Coerulea." *Pharmacology, Biochemistry and Behavior* Vol. 47 (1994): 1–4.

Worgul, T. J., et al. "Evidence That Brain Aromatization Regulates LH Secretions in the Male Dog." *American Journal of Physiology* vol. 241, *Endocrinology Metabolism* vol. 4 (1981): E246–E250.

Wyngaarden, J. B. and L. H. Smith. *Cecil's Textbook of Medicine.* Philadelphia, PA: Saunders, 1985.

Yen, S. S., et al. "Replacement of DHEA in Aging Men and Women: Potential Remedial Effects." *Annals of New York Academy of Science* Vol. 774 (1995): 128–142.

Index

About the Authors

Frederick C. Hatfield holds a Ph.D. in sports science from Temple University. He is president of the International Sports Sciences Association (ISSA), a certifying body and provider of continuing education for personal fitness trainers, health professionals, and strength coaches. He has provided research, development, and marketing consultation to several nutritional and fitness-equipment manufacturers and marketing corporations around the world. He has been involved in, and consultant to, numerous commercial enterprises from the fitness, nutrition, publishing, and education industries since 1970 and has been active in establishing and consulting for numerous health and fitness clubs across the United States. He has taught sports psychology, strength physiology, and physical education at the University of Wisconsin, Newark State College, Bowie State College, University of Illinois, and Temple University. He has been a consultant to the U.S. Olympic Committee, the West German Body Building Federation, Australian Powerlifting Federation, and CBS Sports. He was coach of the U.S. National Powerlifting team and a member of the executive committees of the U.S. Olympic Weightlifting Federation and U.S. Powerlifting Federation.

The founding editor of *Sports Fitness*, Hatfield has written more than 60 books on sports fitness, weight training, and athletic nutrition. He is a former standout college gymnast and a former Mr. Atlantic Coast and Mr. Mid-America in bodybuilding. A former Connecticut State weightlifting champion, he has broken more than 30 world records in five different powerlifting weight divisions, and won world championships in powerlifting three times in three different weight divisions. In 1987, at age 45, Hatfield established a world record in the squat at 1,014 pounds (body weight 255), the most anyone had lifted in the history of competition. His frequent world record–breaking performances have gained him the nickname "Dr. Squat."

Frederick C. Hatfield II, M.S., received his master's degree in sports sciences from Middle Tennessee State University in 1994, where he also served as an assistant strength coach. Prior to that he received his bachelor's degree in exercise physiology from Kent State University. He has competed in powerlifting in the 148-pound and 165-pound weight divisions for the past 12 years. He was the assistant speed, strength, and conditioning coach at James Madison University from 1995 to 1996 and was assistant speed, strength, and conditioning coach at the University of Massachusetts in Amherst from 1996 to 1998. He serves as special projects director and lecturer for the International Sports Sciences Association.